Strengthening Systems to Prevent Intimate Partner Violence and Sexual Violence

Over the past 25 years, developing coordinated responses to intimate partner violence and sexual violence has improved both perpetrator accountability and victim safety and self-determination. However, preventing intimate partner violence and sexual violence from occurring is beyond the ability of any one type of organization. Preventing this violence requires a network of individuals, groups and organizations who coordinate and assess their efforts on an ongoing basis.

This volume provides theoretical and practical guidance for the development of state and local prevention systems that hold the potential to eliminate persistent social problems. The development of prevention systems was informed by the data-driven public health model, systems theory and the ecological systems perspective. *Strengthening Systems to Prevent Intimate Partner Violence and Sexual Violence* offers guidance on how to gain participation of the right partners in developing a prevention system, and how to focus the work of that system on the critical areas of planning, implementation and capacity building. The guidance, resources and experience shared in this important collection will be invaluable to all those working towards the prevention of intimate partner violence and sexual violence.

This book is based on a special issue of the *Journal of Family Social Work.*

Pat Conway is a Senior Research Scientist at the Essentia Institute of Rural Health in Duluth, Minnesota, USA. She is Editor of the *Journal of Family Social Work.*

Pamela J. Cox is a behavioural scientist within the Division of Violence Prevention at the Centers for Disease Control and Prevention in Atlanta, Georgia, USA.

Patricia G. Cook-Craig is Associate Professor in the College of Social Work at the University of Kentucky, Lexington, USA. Her research interests include evaluation of violence prevention planning processes and intervention strategies.

Sandra Ortega is an Independent Consultant for Ohio's DELTA and RPE projects. She conducts program evaluation in education, health and human services throughout the State of Ohio, USA.

Theresa L. Armstead is a behavioural scientist within the Division of Violence Prevention at the Centers for Disease Control and Prevention in Atlanta, Georgia, USA.

Strengthening Systems to Prevent Intimate Partner Violence and Sexual Violence

Edited by
Pat Conway, Pamela J. Cox,
Patricia G. Cook-Craig, Sandra Ortega
and Theresa L. Armstead

Routledge
Taylor & Francis Group
LONDON AND NEW YORK

First published 2013
by Routledge
2 Park Square, Milton Park, Abingdon, Oxfordshire OX14 4RN

Simultaneously published in the USA and Canada
by Routledge
711 Third Avenue, New York, NY 10017

First issued in paperback 2014

Routledge is an imprint of the Taylor & Francis Group, an informa business

This book is a reproduction of *Journal of Family Social Work*, volume 13, issue 4. The Publisher requests to those authors who may be citing this book to state, also, the bibliographical details of the special issue on which the book was based.

British Library Cataloguing in Publication Data
A catalogue record for this book is available from the British Library

ISBN 978-0-415-52288-5 (hbk)
ISBN 978-1-138-84185-7 (pbk)

Typeset in Garamond
by Saxon Graphics

Publisher's Note
The publisher would like to make readers aware that the chapters in this book may be referred to as articles as they are identical to the articles published in the special issue. The publisher accepts responsibility for any inconsistencies that may have arisen in the course of preparing this volume for print.

Contents

Citation Information

The following chapters were originally published in the *Journal of Family Social Work*, volume 13, issue 4 (2010). When citing this material, please use the original page numbering for each article, as follows:

Chapter 3
The Rape Prevention and Education (RPE) Theory Model of Community Change: Connecting Individual and Social Change
Pamela J. Cox, Karen S. Lang, Stephanie M. Townsend and Rebecca Campbell
Journal of Family Social Work, volume 13, issue 4 (2010) pp. 297-312

Chapter 4
Using Social Network Theory to Influence the Development of State and Local Primary Prevention Capacity-Building Teams
Patricia G. Cook-Craig
Journal of Family Social Work, volume 13, issue 4 (2010) pp. 313-325

Chapter 5
Building the Capacity of States to Ensure Inclusion of Rural Communities in State and Local Primary Violence Prevention Planning
Patricia G. Cook-Craig, Karen G. Lane and Wendi L. Siebold
Journal of Family Social Work, volume 13, issue 4 (2010) pp. 326-342

Chapter 6
Using Empowerment Evaluation to Facilitate the Development of Intimate Partner and Sexual Violence Prevention Programs
Pat Conway, Janet Cresswell, Diane Harmon, Charles Pospishil, Kathy Smith, Jennifer Wages and Lisa Weisz
Journal of Family Social Work, volume 13, issue 4 (2010) pp. 343-361

Chapter 7
Youth Action Strategies in the Primary Prevention of Teen Dating Violence
Denise Kervin and Jennifer Obinna
Journal of Family Social Work, volume 13, issue 4 (2010) pp. 362-374

Chapter 8
Changes in Capacity Among Local Coordinated Community Response Coalitions (CCRs) Supported by the DELTA Program
Pamela J. Cox, Daniel M. Finkelstein, Victoria E. Perez and Margo L. Rosenbach
Journal of Family Social Work, volume 13, issue 4 (2010) pp. 375-392

CDC's DELTA and EMPOWER Programs: Strengthening Systems for Primary Prevention of Intimate Partner Violence and Sexual Violence

PAT CONWAY

Essentia Institute of Rural Health, Duluth, MN

PAMELA J. COX AND THERESA L. ARMSTEAD

Centers for Disease Control and Prevention, Atlanta, GA

SANDRA ORTEGA

Independent Consultant for Ohio's DELTA and RPE Programs, Columbus, OH

PATRICIA G. COOK-CRAIG

University of Kentucky, Lexington, KY

The findings and conclusions in this report are those of the authors and do not necessarily represent the official position of the Centers for Disease Control and Prevention.

INTRODUCTION

The Centers for Disease Control and Prevention (2005a, 2005b) has implemented two programs to reduce intimate partner and sexual violence, the DELTA (Domestic Violence Prevention Enhancements and Leadership Through Alliances) Program in 2002 and the EMPOWER (Enhancing and Making Programs Work to End Rape) Program in 2005 (http://www.cdc.gov/ViolencePrevention/FundedPrograms/index.html). Both DELTA and EMPOWER make use of prevention systems defined as networks of individuals, groups, and organizations that, through their interactions, have the potential to enhance the primary prevention of intimate partner violence (IPV) and sexual violence (SV) using a public health approach (Gerteis, Lang, Rosenbach, Finkelstein, Morzuh, Cashman, & Cox, 2010). Systems theory and the ecological systems perspective that individual, family, and community well-being is shaped by the systems that surround them supports the concept of prevention systems (Payne, 2005).

The public health approach employed by the DELTA and EMPOWER Programs complements the use of prevention systems. The public health approach provides a structured, data-driven process for assessing and promoting both individual and environmental changes that can prevent the initial occurrence of IPV and SV (Saltzman, Green, Marks, & Thacker, 2000). The approach uses data to (1) assess how many people are affected by these types of violence in a state or community; (2) identify risk and protective factors, whether individual, relationship, community, or societal; (3) evaluate strategies that target these risk and protective factors; and (4) promote widespread use of strategies that are proven to be effective.

The Centers for Disease Control and Prevention (CDC) defines IPV as physical violence, sexual violence, threats of physical or sexual violence, and psychological/emotional abuse that occur between current or former intimate partners (Saltzman, Fanslow, McMahon, & Shelley, 1999). CDC also recognizes that IPV exists on a continuum from a single episode to ongoing battering, where battering refers to one partner seeking to develop and maintain power and control over the other partner (CDC, 2006; Johnson, 1995). CDC defines SV as a range of behaviors from forced intercourse, to attempted intercourse, to non-contact sexual abuse (e.g., sexual harassment) (Basile & Saltzman, 2002). CDC's key criteria in defining any one or all of these behaviors as SV is whether or not consent to engage in the behavior was freely given by both parties.

Unfortunately, IPV and SV occur frequently in the United States. More than 1 in 3 women and more than 1 in 4 men have experienced rape, physical violence, and/or stalking by an intimate partner in their lifetime (Black, Basile, Breiding, Smith, Walters, Merrick, Chen, & Stevens, 2011). Women and women of color, especially American Indian Alaska Native and multiracial women, experience higher rates of violence (p. 20, p. 39). These statistics illustrate why solutions to prevent IPV and SV before first time occurrence are critical. DELTA and EMPOWER present two programs designed to strengthen prevention systems using a public health approach.

DELTA AND EMPOWER: STRENGTHENING PREVENTION SYSTEMS

The power of a prevention system lies in its ability to promote a sustained, comprehensive and coordinated approach by a network of individuals, groups, and organizations. The complex, socially entrenched nature of IPV and SV require a commensurate comprehensive approach in contrast to a simplistic or uncoordinated approach of increasing funding to independently-operated local shelters and rape crisis centers. The DELTA and EMPOWER Programs address the comprehensive nature of prevention system work through eight dimensions: the System Profile; Leadership; Strategic Planning; Information; Community and Constituency Focus; Human Resources; System Operations; and Results/Outcomes (Gerteis, Lang, Rosenbach, Finkelstein, Morzuh, Cashman, & Cox, 2010). This book presents examples of these more complex solutions, describing models for change, methods for evaluating prevention systems, and strategies employed by those prevention systems.

Through the first dimension, System Profiles, the DELTA and EMPOWER Programs identify key stakeholders and define existing environment, relationships and challenges of their current prevention system (Gerteis, et al., 2010). The Leadership and Strategic Planning dimensions establish priorities for IPV and SV prevention and utilize the credibility and clout of key stakeholders to advance these priorities. The Information dimension promotes the use of data throughout the system to inform decision-making in the areas of planning, formative evaluation, and process evaluation. A Community and Constituency Focus ensures that the prevention system's work is representative of key IPV and SV constituencies. The Human Resources dimension promotes the development of a diverse, well-trained, stable workforce. The Systems Operations dimension includes key prevention programs, strategies, and policies focusing on prevention of IPV and/or SV. Through this dimension, organizations implementing prevention programs, strategies and policies receive implementation and evaluation support focused on improving the organization's ability to achieve its intended outcomes. The final dimension, Results/Outcomes, promotes the use of data to demonstrate short and long-term outcomes. By strengthening these eight dimensions, states and communities work toward the social change needed to prevent the initial occurrence of IPV and SV.

Through the DELTA Program's funding, training, and technical assistance, CDC supports 14 state domestic violence coalitions in Alaska, California, Delaware, Florida, Kansas, Michigan, Montana, New York, North Carolina, North Dakota, Ohio, Rhode Island, Virginia, and Wisconsin. A unique characteristic of the DELTA Program was an explicit emphasis on strengthening local-level prevention systems through its support of a coordinated community responses (CCR). Within the DELTA Program, a CCR was defined as an organized effort representing diverse sectors of a local community that addresses IPV by integrating prevention and intervention strategies and services through increased communication, cooperation, and coordination (CDC, 2005a). CCRs often operate as informal, unincorporated community coalitions, in which a group of organizations and individuals who have common interests work toward achieving common goals (Florin, Mitchell, & Stevenson, 1993). As of January 2010, 59 CCRs were supported by the DELTA state domestic violence coalitions.

The EMPOWER Program, an enhancement of CDC's nation-wide SV prevention program, the Rape Prevention and Education (RPE) Program. RPE supports the SV prevention efforts of health departments in all 50 states and 9 U.S. territories. The EMPOWER Program supports a subset of RPE grantees (Colorado, Kentucky, New Jersey, Massachusetts, North Carolina, and North Dakota) with additional funding, training, and technical assistance specifically focused on state-level data-driven planning, implementation, evaluation and sustainability efforts.

Both the DELTA and EMPOWER Programs required each state to develop a comprehensive state plan to provide a blueprint for a coordinated approach to IPV and SV prevention. State plans were to be data-driven and support the use of the best available research evidence to identify and choose strategies for groups at most risk for experiencing IPV and SV. One distinctive feature of the plans was a complementary assessment of each state's prevention system, so that the weakest dimensions of their coordinated approach could be identified and addressed.

To facilitate the development of state plans, CDC needed a planning framework and an evaluation approach that would integrate well with the values and perspectives of key DELTA and EMPOWER Program stakeholders and would appeal to feminist and grassroots perspectives held by many people and organizations that have long worked to end IPV and SV (Sloan, 2006). CDC chose to adapt Getting To Outcomes (Chinman, Imm, Wandersman, 2004) due to its reputation in the substance abuse field as a practitioner-friendly planning, evaluation and sustainability model that easily integrates grassroots concerns and experiences. Based on the first six steps of Getting to Outcomes, the DELTA and EMPOWER Programs completed a state-wide needs and resources assessment; developed goals and outcomes; chose strategies; assessed compatibility; assessed capacity, and finalized their plans (Chinman, Imm, Wandersman, 2004).

CDC chose an empowerment evaluation approach for the DELTA and EMPOWER Programs, due to empowerment evaluation's grounding in 10 principles that reflect many of the feminist principles held by key DELTA and EMPOWER stakeholders within each state: improvement, community ownership, inclusion, democratic participation, social justice, community knowledge, evidence-based strategies, capacity building, organizational learning, and accountability (Wandersman, et al., 2005). Each DELTA and EMPOWER state was required to hire an empowerment evaluator. Under this approach, these evaluators were not an authority who did the planning or formative evaluation work and then presented the work to stakeholders for review, comment, and adoption. Instead, evaluators utilized the 10 empowerment evaluation principles to facilitate a learn-by-doing process, whereby DELTA and EMPOWER stakeholders conducted their own data-driven planning process and increased their capacities to conduct such work in the future (Cox, Keener, Woodard, & Wandersman, 2009).

To develop the state plan in a manner that reflected the 10 empowerment evaluation principles, each DELTA and EMPOWER state organized state steering committees or state prevention teams respectively. The groups were comprised of diverse agencies, organizations, and individuals. A three member capacity-building team guided the state-level prevention committee/team through the planning process. Two key members of the capacity building team were the DELTA/EMPOWER coordinator and the empowerment evaluator. The third member was the executive director of the state domestic violence coalition for DELTA or a state prevention team member in EMPOWER.

The coordinated approach of DELTA coalitions, the EMPOWER Programs' health departments, state steering committees and prevention teams, empowerment evaluators; and the CDC provides a model where stakeholders work together for primary prevention of Intimate Partner Violence. Lessons learned provide guidance for others seeking to build momentum for primary prevention in their community.

SUMMARY OF CHAPTERS

This book presents the theories undergirding the two programs, examples of application of the programs, and capacity building at the state and local level. The first two chapters cover the history and theory behind the DELTA and EMPOWER Programs.

Theresa L. Armstead, Pamela J. Cox, Daniel M. Finkelstein and Margo L. Rosenbach set the stage for the DELTA Program and gives the history of intimate partner violence, in "The Primary Prevention Work of State Domestic Violence Coalitions Supported by the Domestic Violence Prevention Enhancements and Leadership Through Alliances (DELTA) Program." The authors then present the results of a survey of state domestic violence coalitions' general and prevention capacity and their initial prevention activities.

"The Rape Prevention and Education (RPE) Theory Model of Community Change: Connecting Individual and Social Change," by Pamela Cox, Karen Lang, Stephanie Townsend and Rebecca Campbell, cover the RPE Theory Model of Community Change, which utilizes the theories of Community Readiness, Diffusion of Innovation, Theory of Reasoned Action and the Health Belief Model. An example of its application to state-level SV prevention planning, the New Jersey EMPOWER Program, demonstrates how individuals and communities change separately and concurrently. Both the theoretical concepts and New Jersey case example highlight the need to develop broad-based, diverse partnerships and community readiness for the type of social and systems change that will eventually lead to the prevention of SV.

The next four chapters describe DELTA and EMPOWER program implementation in four states. Patty Cook-Craig, in "Using Social Network Theory to Influence the Development of State and Local Primary Prevention Capacity Building Teams", examines social network theory's contribution to the development of the Kentucky EMPOWER Program's state-level primary prevention plan. The author reviews the assumptions of social network theory that were useful in guiding the planning process. Using social network analysis visualization techniques, Cook-Craig outlines how prevention partners in communities across Kentucky varied in the way that they networked together and discusses implications for how networking differences influenced the planning process in these communities.

"Building the Capacity of States to Ensure Inclusion of Rural Communities in State and Local Primary Violence Prevention Planning" by Patty Cook-Craig, Karen Lane, and Wendi Seibold, describes challenges that the rural nature of Kentucky and Montana created in promoting and planning primary prevention.

They present strategies that encouraged active involvement and representation by rural communities in each state's planning process.

Pat Conway, Diane Harmon, Charles Pospishil, Kathy Smith, Jennifer Wages, Lisa Weisz, and Janet Cresswell present three case studies of local communities that successfully implemented the first step of their IPV and/or SV prevention work: the completion of a needs and resource assessment. "Using Empowerment Evaluation to Facilitate the Development of Intimate Partner and Sexual Violence Prevention Programs" identifies factors that contributed to each community's success and ways in which challenges were addressed. The insights offered through the data collection examples and their associated challenges and analysis of organizational, community, state, and national factors leading to successful completion of the needs assessments demonstrate the utility of the empowerment evaluation process. The lessons learned can be applied in other communities to further inform the question about the impact the empowerment evaluation process has on developing successful prevention programs.

Denise Kervin and Jennifer Obinna detail the work of a rural Wisconsin DELTA CCR in "Youth Action Strategies in the Primary Prevention of Teen Dating Violence." The authors describe a youth-led health approach to teen dating violence that provides an excellent opportunity for youth to become involved and empowered to create social change within a school setting. A partnership between the program's designers, schools, students, teachers and school social workers was leveraged to build a foundation of knowledge about how to produce social change and a structure that appeals to and obtains buy-in from its participants. The article elucidates the transformation of the project participants and the program over four years of implementation, offering lessons learned for replication elsewhere.

The final chapter, "Changes in Capacity among Local Coordinated Community Response Coalitions Supported by the DELTA Program," reviews the 59 local DELTA CCRs' progress in developing capacities and utilizing supports needed by coalitions to effectively address IPV and SV. Pamela Cox, Daniel Finklestein, Victoria Perez, and Margo Rosenbach examine the progress of local coalitions through the Interactive Systems Framework for Dissemination and Implementation (ISF), which provides a glimpse of the substantial infrastructure needed to effectively work toward social change and ultimately the prevention of IPV. One key lesson is that the integration of primary prevention within coalitions that have historically focused on intervention can be done, but it takes time and dedicated effort.

THE POTENTIAL OF PREVENTION SYSTEMS

The development of prevention systems focusing on primary prevention of IPV and SV holds the potential to eliminate these persistent social problems. Based on the experiences of the DELTA and EMPOWER Programs, this book provides theoretical and practical guidance on ways to develop state and local prevention systems. Although the assumption is that a coordinated prevention system is greater than the sum of its parts, this holds true only under two conditions. The first condition is that the right parts, or partners, are brought into the system, and the second condition is that the system must engage in substantive rather than superficial efforts to address important individual and environmental risk and protective factors. This book offers guidance on methods for gaining participation by the right partners when developing a prevention system and how to focus the work of the system on the critical areas of planning, implementation, and capacity building. This guidance can save other states and communities valuable time, effort, and resources in their efforts to prevent IPV and SV.

REFERENCES

Basile K. C., Chen J., Black, M. C., & Saltzman, L. E., (2007) Prevalence and characteristics of sexual violence victimization among U.S. adults, 2001-2003. *Violence and Victims, 22*, 437-448.

Basile, K. C., & Saltzman, L. E. (2002). *Sexual violence surveillance: Uniform definitions and recommended data elements.* Atlanta, GA: National Center for Injury Prevention and Control, Centers for Disease Control and Prevention.

Black, M. C., Basile, K. C., Breiding, M. J., Smith, S. G., Walters, M. L., Merrick, M. T., Chen, J., & Stevens, M. R. (2011). *The National Intimate Partner and Sexual Violence Survey*. Atlanta, Georgia: Centers for Disease Control and Prevention.

Campbell, J. C., & Soeken, K. L. (1999). Forced sex and intimate partner violence. *Violence Against Women, 5*, 1017-1035.

Centers for Disease Control and Prevention. (2006). *Understanding intimate partner violence fact sheet.* Retrieved May 1, 2009, from National Center for Disease Control and Prevention Web site: http://www.cdc.gov/ViolencePrevention/pdf/IPV-FactSheet.pdf

Centers for Disease Control and Prevention. (2005a). Domestic violence prevention enhancement and leadership through alliances (DELTA) Program: Funding Opportunity Number: RFA 05039. Federal Register / Vol. 70, No. 37 / Friday, February 25, 2005 / Notices, pages 9320-9329.

Centers for Disease Control and Prevention. (2005b). Building comprehensive prevention program planning and evaluation capacity for rape prevention and education funded programs: Funding opportunity number: 05037. Federal Register /Vol. 70, No. 51/ Thursday, March 17, 2005 /Notices. Pages 130333 – 130337

Chinman, M., Imm, P., & Wandersman, A., (2004). *Getting to Outcomes: Promoting accountability through methods and tools for planning, implementation and evaluation.* Santa Monica, CA: Rand Corporation.

Cook-Craig, P. (2010). Using social network theory to influence the development of state and local primary prevention capacity building teams. *Journal of Family Social Work, 13* (4), 313-325.

Cook-Craig, P. Lane, K., & Seibold, W. (2010). Building the capacity of states to ensure inclusion of rural communities in state and local primary violence prevention planning. *Journal of Family Social Work, 13* (4), 326-342.

Conway, P., Pospishil, M., Wages, J., Harmon, K., Smith, N., & Weiz, R. (2010). Using empowerment evaluation to facilitate the development of intimate partner and sexual violence prevention programs. *Journal of Family Social Work, 13* (4), 343-361.

Cox, P. J., Finkelstein, D. M., Perez, V. E., Rosenback, M. L., (2010). Changes in capacity among local coordinated community response coalitions supported by the DELTA Program. *Journal of Family Social Work, 13* (4), 375-392.

Cox, P. J., Keener D., Woodard, T., & Wandersman A. (2009). *Evaluation for improvement: a seven step empowerment evaluation approach for violence prevention organizations.* Atlanta, GA: Centers for Disease Control and Prevention.

Cox, P. J., Lang, K., Townsend, S., & Campbell, R. (2010). The rape prevention and education (RPE) theory model of community change: Connecting individual and social change. *Journal of Family Social Work, 13* (4), 297-312.

Florin, P., Mitchell, R., & Stevenson, J. (1993). Identifying training and technical assistance needs in community coalitions: A developmental approach. *Health Education Research: Theory and Practice, 8*, 417-432.

Gerteis, M., Lang, K. S., Rosenbach, M., Finkelstein, D., Morzuh, M., Cashman, S., & Cox, P. (2010). System capacity for sexual violence prevention within states: Lessons from the cross-site evaluation of enhancing and making programs and outcomes work to end rape (EMPOWER).

Hobart, M. (1998). *Homicide at home: Washington State's domestic violence fatality review project.* Seattle, WA: Washington State Coalition Against Domestic Violence. Retrieved April 30, 2010, from Washington State Coalition Against Domestic Violence Web site: http://www.wscadv.org/resourcesPublications.cfm?aId=825E4311-C298-58F6-0193BC0320EDBA58

Johnson, M. P. (1995). Patriarchal terrorism and common couple violence: Two forms of violence against women in U.S. families. *Journal of Marriage and the Family, 57*, 283-294.

Kervin, D. & Obinna, J. (2010). Youth action strategies in the primary prevention of teen dating violence. *Journal of Family Social Work, 13* (4), 362-374.

McDonald, R., Jouriles, E. N., Ramisetty-Mikler, S., Caetano, R., & Green, C. E. (2006). Estimating the number of American children living in partner-violent families. *Journal of Family Psychology, 20*(1), 137-142.

National Association of Social Workers (2005). *NASW standards for clinical social work in social work practices.* Washington, DC: National Association of Social Workers.

Payne, M. (2005). Systems and ecological perspectives. *Modern social work theory (3rd ed)* (pp.142-160). Chicago: Lyceum Books.

Saltzman, L. E., Fanslow, J. L., McMahon, P. M., & Shelley, G.A. (1999). *Intimate partner violence surveillance: Uniform definitions and recommended data elements, Version 1.0.* Atlanta, GA: National Center for Injury Prevention and Control, Centers for Disease Control and Prevention.

Saltzman, L. E., Greene, Y. T., Marks, J. S., & Thacker, S. B., (2000). Violence against women as a public health issue: Comments from the CDC. *American Journal of Preventive Medicine, 19*(4), 325-329.

Sloan, L. M. (2006). Two movements, two paths, one goal. *Revolution 1*, 3-6. Retrieved April 30, 2010, from Virginia Sexual and Domestic Violence Action Alliance Web site: http://www.vadv.org/secPublications/Revolution%201-Winter2006pages1-11.pdf

Stout, K. D., & McPhail, B. (1998). *Confronting sexism and violence against women: A challenge for social work*. New York, NY: Longman.

U.S. Department of Justice. (2010). Homicide trends in the U.S.: Intimate homicide. Retrieved March 24, 2010, from Bureau of Justice Statistics Web site: http://bjs.ojp.usdoj.gov/content/homicide/tables/intimatestab.cfm

Wandersman, A., Snell-Johns, J., Lentz, B. E., Fetterman, D. M., Keener, D. C., Livet, M., Imm, P. S., & Flaspohler, P. (2005). The principles of empowerment evaluation. In D. M. Fetterman & A. Wandersmand (Eds.), *Empowerment evaluation principles in practice* (pp. 27-41). New York: Guilford Press.

The Primary Prevention Work of State Domestic Violence Coalitions Supported by the Domestic Violence Prevention Enhancements and Leadership Through Alliances (DELTA) Program

THERESA L. ARMSTEAD AND PAMELA J. COX
Centers for Disease Control and Prevention

DANIEL M. FINKELSTEIN AND MARGO L. ROSENBACH
Mathematica Policy Research

The Centers for Disease Control and Prevention (CDC) recognizes that the elimination of intimate partner violence (IPV) will require building the capacity among practitioner organizations to prevent the initial occurrence of IPV. The practice of IPV primary prevention is currently in its formative stage. This chapter describes the history of the service and advocacy work of the State Domestic Violence Coalitions (SDVCs), organizations in which primary prevention is being integrated by the CDC DELTA Program. Further, this chapter uses evaluation data from CDC's DELTA Program to show the variety of ways 14 SDVCs have built IPV primary prevention capacity within their organizations. The findings highlight the importance of tailoring capacity-building activities to each state's unique circumstances and not assuming a "one-size-fits-all" approach to the primary prevention of IPV.

The Centers for Disease Control and Prevention (CDC) defines intimate partner violence (IPV) as physical violence, sexual violence, threats of physical or sexual violence, and psychological/emotional abuse that occurs between current or former intimate partners (Saltzman, Fanslow, McMahon, & Shelley, 1999). IPV exists on a continuum from a single episode to ongoing battering (i.e., domestic violence) (CDC, 2006; Johnson, 1995), in which battering refers to one partner seeking to develop and maintain power and control over the other. IPV is a serious public health problem in the United States. More than 1 in 3 women and more than 1 in 4 men have experienced rape, physical violence, and/or stalking by an intimate partner in their lifetime (Black, Basile, Breiding, Smith, Walters, Merrick, Chen, & Stevens, 2011). Efforts that attempt to prevent first-time perpetration or first-time victimization of IPV are primary prevention; efforts that respond to cases of IPV are interventions, or secondary and tertiary prevention (Dahlberg & Krug, 2002).

Over the past 30 years, the United States has made significant advances in IPV intervention efforts, such as developing shelters for victims and their children; creating battering intervention programs for perpetrators; changing criminal laws, policies, and practices that promote victim safety and self-determination and offender accountability; providing civil law remedies for victims; and expanding medical screening and referral for victims. State Domestic Violence Coalitions (SDVCs) began conceptualizing, advocating for, disseminating, and implementing advances in IPV intervention in the late 1970's and early 1980s. However, advances in IPV intervention strategies across the United States have not been matched with advances in primary prevention strategies that serve to change the underlying protective and risk factors that reduce the likelihood of IPV. To strengthen attention to primary prevention, in 2002 CDC's Domestic Violence Prevention Enhancements and Leadership Through Alliances (DELTA) Program funded nine SDVCs to advance the primary prevention of IPV within their respective states by building the SDVCs' general (i.e., organizational) and prevention capacities. In 2003, CDC funded five more SDVCs to bring the total to 14: Alaska, California, Delaware, Florida, Kansas, Michigan, Montana, New York, North Carolina, North Dakota, Ohio, Rhode Island, Virginia, and Wisconsin. Throughout this chapter DELTA Program SDVCs will refer to these listed states only.

In 2002, CDC initiated the DELTA Program in accordance with the year 2000 authorizing legislation: Section 10418 of the Family Violence Prevention and Services Act (FVSPA) (2002), Demonstration Grants for Community Initiatives. The purpose of the DELTA Program was to integrate primary prevention principles, concepts, and practices into local coordinated community responses (CCRs), a type of local community coalition that has traditionally focused on how to intervene in or respond to cases of IPV (Department of Health and Human Services – Centers for Disease Control and Prevention [DHHS-CDC], 2005). CDC wanted to build on existing infrastructures to promote the successful integration of primary prevention within the CCR model. In assessing the infrastructure of the field, CDC noted that SDVCs had statewide IPV-related training and technical assistance infrastructures, which were available to CCRs. As a result of the assessment, CDC decided to fund SDVCs to provide primary prevention-focused training, technical assistance, and funding to local CCRs. As of April 2012, the DELTA Program SDVCs supported approximately 45 local CCRs (CDC, 2011).

This chapter has two purposes: to provide a historical foundation for the integration of primary prevention capacity building into the traditional work of SDVCs and to report on the primary prevention capacities and activities of the DELTA Program SDVCs based on the DELTA Program's evaluation data. To achieve the first purpose, this chapter provides a brief historical overview of the development of SDVCs. Specifically, the chapter describes their historical work in two core areas, social change (e.g., legislative reforms) and intervention (e.g., supporting organizations that address the needs of victims of IPV), and grounds the historical work within the Interactive Systems Framework for Dissemination and Implementation (ISF) (Wandersman et al., 2008).

Conceptually, the ISF is a research-to-practice framework that illustrates the movement of effective prevention practices, programs, and/or principles through a set of systematically or coherently organized activities; termed *systems* in this framework. The ISF has three systems: prevention synthesis and translation, prevention support, and prevention delivery. In this chapter the ISF is being used to provide a conceptual framework for understanding the DELTA SDVCs' primary prevention activity and the capacities needed to support the work (see Wandersman et al., 2008 for a detailed description of the three systems). This modified application of the ISF frames movement of research knowledge through the prevention systems when effective strategies are not available.

OVERVIEW OF STATE DOMESTIC VIOLENCE COALITIONS

For the purposes of this chapter, the term *State Domestic Violence Coalition* (SDVC) refers to organizations that receive grant funds under Section 10410 of the Family Violence Prevention Services Act (FVPSA; 1994), Grants for State Domestic Violence Coalitions. Since 1994, this section of the FVPSA has directed the U.S. Department of Health and Human Services to provide grants to SDVCs that:

1. Are statewide nonprofit organizations.
2. Have memberships that are representative of the majority of the organizations that serve victims of IPV within their respective states.
3. Have boards of directors that are representative of such organizations.
4. Provide services, community education, and technical assistance to organizations that provide services to victims of IPV and their children regarding the implementation and operation of shelters and related services.

As of the 2010 reauthorization, all 50 states, the District of Columbia, the Commonwealth of Puerto Rico, Guam, Northern Mariana Islands, American Samoa, and the Virgin Islands have SDVCs that receive FVPSA funding (National Network to End Domestic Violence [NNEDV], n.d.).

HISTORY OF SDVCS

The earliest SDVCs were established in the late 1970s, and the most recently formed SDVCs were established in the early 1990s. For example, the New York State Coalition Against Domestic Violence was initiated in 1978, while the Delaware Coalition Against Domestic Violence was founded in 1994 (New York

State Coalition Against Domestic Violence, 2008; Delaware Coalition Against Domestic Violence, 2004). Many state coalitions started out as informal networks of local organizations that served victims of IPV and over time transitioned to become formal, 501(c)3, nonprofit organizations that represented the needs of their member organizations (Florida Coalition Against Domestic Violence, n.d., North Dakota Council on Abused Women's Services, n.d.). Today, many SDVCs have various categories of membership, such as private, nonprofit organizations that serve victims of IPV and their children, allied organizations, and individual members (NNEDV, 2007).

Although SDVCs grew out of the battered women's movement in the United States, each SDVC has a unique history, operating structure, political context, funding structure, and set of priorities (NNEDV, 2007; Schechter, 1982). Two major commonalities among SDVCs are that they consider their ultimate constituency to be victims of IPV and that their membership is mainly composed of organizations that address the needs of IPV victims (e.g., organizations that provide shelter services). Thus, SDVCs have focused their work in two core areas: social change work that benefits all victims of IPV (NNEDV, 2007) and intervention work that directly or indirectly supports victims of IPV who seek services (NNEDV, 2007; Schechter, 1982). Despite their important role in advancing IPV intervention efforts over the past 30 years, the work of SDVCs has not been thoroughly examined or well documented in the peer-reviewed literature.

SDVCS WORK AND THE INTERACTIVE SYSTEMS FRAMEWORK (ISF)

The work of SDVCs involves social change, intervention, and prevention activities. SDVCs' intervention and prevention activities can be organized within a modified application of the three systems of the Interactive Systems Framework for Dissemination and Implementation (ISF): synthesis and translation; prevention support; and prevention delivery. Originally, the ISF was developed to move effective innovations into practice, but it is a dissemination framework that is also applicable to moving intervention and prevention strategies based on the best available research knowledge into practice. Therefore, the three ISF systems are used to illustrate the activities that facilitate widespread adoption of the intervention and prevention practices that are based on the best available evidence (Figure 1).

The synthesis and translation system frames how effective practices for both intervention and prevention are synthesized and translated for use by various practitioners. The support system frames how activities, such as training and technical assistance, are needed to support practitioners adopting best practices after synthesis and translation. The delivery system frames implementation of best practices to prevent or reduce the occurrence of IPV. Figure 1 also depicts SDVCs' social change activities (e.g., reforms at local, state, and national levels), which are outside the scope of the original ISF but are at the very heart of what SDVCs do.

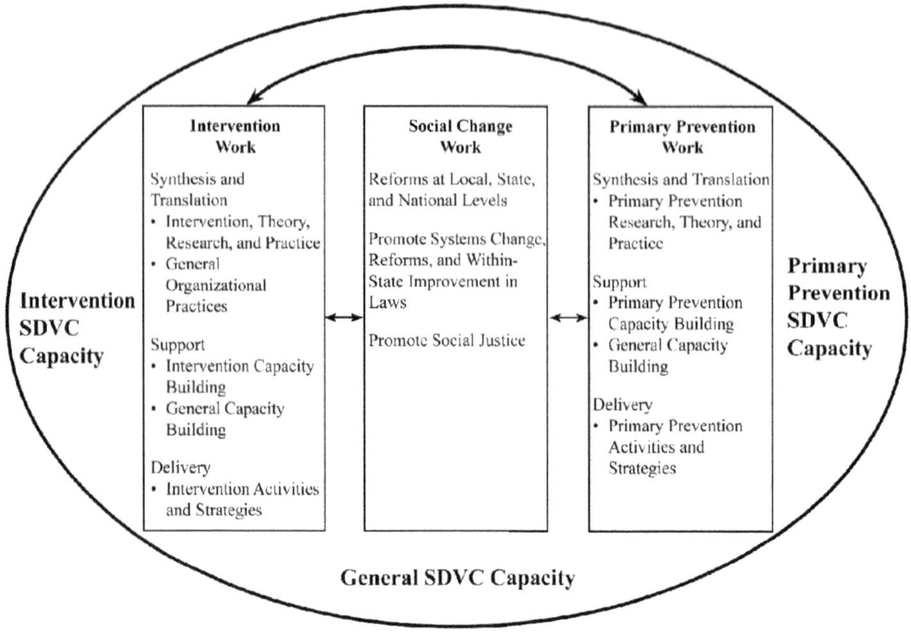

FIGURE 1 Activities of the DELTA Program State Domestic Violence Coalitions (SDVC)

SDVCs have contributed to *social change work* by creating awareness about IPV and the resources, programming, services, and leadership that are necessary to reduce IPV. This work informs within-state systems change, reforms, and changes in laws and promotes social justice. Specifically, Section 10402 of FVPSA (2007) requires state FVPSA administrators (i.e., the designated state government agency) to establish procedures for including SDVCs in the planning and implementation of their FVPSA grant. The U.S. Department of Health and Human Services Administration on Children and Families provides more explicit guidance (n.d.) to state FVPSA administrators that requires them to ensure that SDVCs "play a meaningful role in identifying eligible organizations and activities, determining how to equitably distribute funds to programs across the state, and determining underserved populations" (p. 18). Thus, this support at all levels of government provides SDVCs with a platform through which to substantially promote within-state systems change and reforms.

The *SDVC intervention work* has *synthesized* information regarding the best intervention and general organizational practices, theory, and research (e.g., statewide public education campaigns and statewide hotlines) (DHHS-ACF, 1995; Schechter, 1982), and *translated* this information into user-friendly formats for organizations that provide direct services to victims of IPV and other audiences. SDVCs have also proactively *supported* local community coalitions and local organizations, such as battered women's shelters (Cox, Finklestein, Perez, & Rosenbach, 2010), in putting this synthesized and translated information into practice through the *delivery* of training and technical assistance offered through site visits, statewide conferences, and regional meetings (DOJ-OVW, 2009; Florida Coalition Against Domestic Violence, n.d.; North Dakota Council on Abused Women's Services, n.d). Additionally, SDVCs have supported local organizations across the state by bringing representatives of member organizations together for informal sharing of successes, challenges, and lessons learned; mutual support; and assistance with building motivation at the state and local levels to address IPV (DHHS-ACF, 1995; DHHS-ACF, 1997; DOJ-OVW, 2009; NNEDV, 2007).

Upon being awarded DELTA Program grants, the DELTA Program SDVCs began integrating *primary prevention work* within their organizations' missions in a manner that built on and was informed by their historical areas of work: social change and intervention. Like the intervention work of SDVCs, the DELTA Program SDVC primary prevention work also includes synthesis and translation, support, and delivery activities (Cox, Finklestein, Perez, & Rosenbach, 2010). DELTA Program SDVCs *synthesize* primary prevention information, such as public health prevention information, theory, and practices that reflect the DELTA Program's emphasis on primary prevention, as well as promising IPV primary prevention practices from within their own states and across the county. The DELTA Program SDVCs *translate* this information into user-friendly products for DELTA-funded CCRs and other audiences (including other state agencies and CCRs not funded by DELTA). The DELTA Program SDVCs provide *support* to the CCRs and other local organizations in developing their primary prevention activities through training and technical assistance using the synthesized and translated information.

The DELTA Program SDVCs' *delivery* activities reflect the DELTA Program's emphasis on primary prevention by (1) reducing risk factors associated with IPV; (2) promoting protective factors that reduce the likelihood of IPV (e.g., behaviors and attitudes associated with healthy intimate relationships); (3) conducting evidence- and theory-supported prevention planning; (4) implementing strategies to address risk and protective factors at all levels of the social ecology (i.e., individual, relationship, community, and societal); and (5) evaluating the effectiveness of primary prevention activities (DHHS-CDC, 2005). These activities reflect the unique contribution of the DELTA Program to the work of SDVCs using the public health approach that emphasizes health promotion.

As Figure 1 further illustrates, to carry out their work DELTA Program SDVCs require *general, intervention, and prevention capacity:* the internal SDVC structures, processes, resources, and leadership that maintain, sustain, and strengthen their abilities to conduct their work. General and prevention capacities are also recognized in the ISF (Wandersman et al, 2008). General capacity supports the SDVCs' ability to implement or improve any program, process, principle, or policy, whether focused on social change, intervention, or prevention (Flaspohler, Duffy, Wandersman, Stillman, & Maras, 2008). *General capacity* may include having written mission statements and/or strategic plans, fiscal management processes, personnel management processes, and sufficient office supplies and equipment. Research suggests that organizations with sufficient general capacity are more able to successfully implement new types of work and activities than organizations without sufficient general capacity (Livet, Courser, & Wandersman, 2008).

SDVC *intervention capacity* supports and sustains intervention work and includes such things as a mission statement that addresses the needs of victims of IPV, training and supervision processes for intervention-oriented work, funding for the intervention, and leadership support. SDVCs have worked with organizations that provide services to victims of IPV to build intervention capacity (e.g., how to operate a shelter) and general capacity (e.g., how to incorporate as private nonprofit organizations) of these organizations so that they may provide victims of IPV with the best services possible (e.g., statewide public education campaigns and statewide hotlines) (DHHS-ACF, 1995, 1997).

Within the DELTA Program, *prevention capacity* is defined as the structures, processes, resources, and leadership support needed by DELTA Program SDVCs to promote and implement the public health model. Additionally the DELTA Program SDVCs proactively build the prevention and general capacity of DELTA-funded CCRs by including the content of synthesized and translated information in DELTA-funded CCR training, technical assistance, and monitoring activities. The specific primary prevention work of the DELTA Program SDVCs will be presented in the next section of this chapter.

FINDINGS FROM AN ASSESSMENT OF THE DELTA PROGRAM

As previously mentioned, advances in IPV prevention (including primary prevention) have not kept up with the significant advances in SDVC social change and intervention work. The CDC DELTA Program was designed to encourage DELTA Program SDVCs to build their general and primary prevention capacity and engage in primary prevention work. The primary prevention synthesis and translation, support, and delivery activities and the general and prevention capacities of the DELTA Program SDVCs were examined in 2006, one year into the three-year program period. Although general capacity is broader than the prevention focus, as described previously in the chapter it is necessary for successfully implementing the primary prevention activity encouraged by the DELTA Program.

METHOD

Organizational Prevention Capacity Questionnaire (OPCQ). The OPCQ was developed by a workgroup comprised of DELTA Program SDVC executive directors, project coordinators, and empowerment evaluators as part of the DELTA Program cross-site evaluation. The questionnaire assessed organizational characteristics relating to the *general capacity* and *prevention capacity* of the coalition (see Table 1). As described in the previous section, general capacity supports a coalition's ability to implement or improve any program, process, principle, or

TABLE 1 Elements of SDVC General and Prevention Capacity

General Capacity	Prevention Capacity
• Total number of full-time equivalent employees • Annual budget • Sources of funding • Frequency of board meetings • Presence of subcommittees • Collaborations with other organizations • Implementation status of organizational structures (e.g., by-laws, written mission statement, strategic plan)	• Number of full-time equivalent employees focused on IPV prevention • Percentage of the annual budget spent on prevention • Sources of funding for prevention • Presence, composition, and activities of an SDVC staff-level prevention team or workgroup • Implementation status of organizational structures for prevention (e.g., job descriptions include prevention, mission statement, strategic plan) • Resources for planning primary prevention activities • Coalitions' efforts to obtain funding to support prevention activities in the future (after DELTA Program funding ends)

policy, whether focused on social change, intervention, or prevention. Prevention capacity is defined as the leadership support, structures, resources, and processes needed by a coalition to promote and implement the public health model. Defined broadly, SDVC leadership refers to both the *formal* leadership provided by the board of directors, the executive director, and others in management positions within the SDVC as well as *informal* leadership provided by other SDVC staff members.

In addition to obtaining information on DELTA Program SDVC general and prevention organizational capacities, the questionnaire assessed the SDVCs' prevention-focused synthesis and translation, support, and delivery activities through both closed- and open-ended questions. For prevention-focused synthesis and translation activities, questions assessed whether or not each DELTA Program SDVC had developed a curriculum reflecting best practices of effective prevention programs (Nation et al., 2003), created guidelines for agencies and organizations involved in primary prevention, and incorporated primary prevention concepts into local trainings. The response options for these items were on a Likert-type scale ranging from 1 to 5, respectively indicating the activity was completed, in process, in planning, under consideration, or not happening at all.

The OPCQ assessed prevention support activities. A list of IPV prevention stakeholders (e.g., colleges and universities) was provided, and DELTA Program SDVCs indicated (i.e., yes, no, or don't know) if support was provided to each group. The DELTA Program SDVCs also reported on how provided support was provided to stakeholders (e.g., conferences, trainings, webcasts, or other), and whether DELTA Program SDVCs used organized methods to evaluate their prevention-focused training and technical assistance activities (i.e., Likert-type scale ranging from fully implemented to no activity at all). The DELTA Program SDVCs also reported on their specific prevention delivery activities, such as planning prevention strategies for priority populations and ensuring that press releases following major IPV incidents included messages about primary prevention. The response options for these items were on a Likert-type scale ranging from 1 to 5, respectively indicating the activity was completed, in process, in planning, under consideration, or not happening at all. To capture prevention work in its broadest sense, the questionnaire provided opportunities for DELTA Program SDVCs to report through open-ended items on other primary prevention synthesis and translation, support, and delivery activities not specifically listed in the survey.

OPCQ administration. In 2007, the DELTA Program SDVCs completed the self-administered OPCQ based on work performed in 2006 in order to assess their early progress toward capacity building. DELTA Project Coordinators at each of the 14 SDVCs completed the survey. Informants were encouraged to use a collaborative process to complete the questionnaire. The collaborative process was designed to solicit input from the SDVCs' executive directors, staff, board members, and empowerment evaluators.

Data analysis. To analyze the information gathered with the OPCQ, descriptive statistics related to the general and prevention capacity and the primary prevention work of the DELTA Program SDVCs were computed. In general, due to the small size of the DELTA program, the number (rather than percentage) of SDVCs with a given attribute is reported. Statistical comparisons across subgroups of coalitions are not presented due to the small number of sites (N=14).

RESULTS

The results section first describes the DELTA Program SDVCs' general capacity and then presents the findings regarding prevention capacity. The results pertain to operating structures, organizational processes, staffing, and resources that contribute to SDVCs' general capacity, prevention capacity, or both. Finally, the results section reports on primary prevention work in the areas of synthesis and translation, support, and delivery.

SDVC General Capacity. The DELTA Program SDVCs reported on governance structures, operating structures, and resources that maintain and enhance their ability to support their prevention activities. All 14 SDVCs reported having a governance structure that included a board of directors. However, the SDVCs reported a wide variation in the size and frequency of meetings for their boards of directors. The median number of board members was 16, ranging from a low of 7 to a high of 36. Nine coalitions had in-person board meetings on a quarterly basis; five met every other month or more frequently. The 14 SDVCs reported 43 different board subcommittees in total, with the most common subcommittees being Finance (10 SDVCs), Executive (9), Development (6), Legislative (5), Membership (4), Personnel (3), Board Development (3), and Certification (3). The median number of subcommittees per SDVC was 5.5, ranging from 2 to 12.

Operating structures for general capacity. Most SDVCs reported having fully implemented the following general operating structures: bylaws/rules of operation (13), written mission statement (12), written staff job descriptions (12), written vision statement (10), a written strategic plan (9), written goals and objectives (8), an organizational chart (8), and minutes recorded on a regular basis at staff meetings (8). The nine SDVCs with written strategic plans reported that their plans were last updated between 2004 and 2007, during the period when SDVCs were receiving DELTA Program funding.

Resources. The 14 DELTA Program SDVCs were supported by multiple funding sources and as a result wide variations in overall funding were reported for 2006. Two SDVCs had an operating budget of more than $3 million, nine had a budget between $1 and $3 million, and three had a budget of less than $1 million. The DELTA Program SDVCs also reported wide variations in the size of their overall staff. In 2006, the median number of full-time equivalent (FTE) employees was 11, ranging from 7 to 25.

SDVC Prevention Capacity. SDVCs reported having developed various prevention capacities that maintain and enhance their prevention work. The number of FTE employees carrying out the prevention work was fairly consistent across the DELTA Program SDVCs. All were required to have one FTE, and three SDVCs reported two or more FTEs for prevention.

Leadership support. The DELTA Program SDVCs varied in their leadership's level of engagement in prevention capacity building and the intensity of prevention planning activities in which leaders participated. With regards to informal leadership, 11 of the 14 DELTA SDVCs reported having a staff-level prevention team to plan and carry out prevention activities in 2006; one SDVC reported having a prevention subcommittee at the board of director's level. The other two SDVCs reported that they did not have an organized group that planned and carried out primary prevention activities. Among the 11 SDVCs with prevention teams, the teams ranged in size from 4 to 8 participants, with a median of 5 participants. All prevention teams included DELTA Program staff, 10 included empowerment evaluators, and nine included the SDVC executive directors and other management staff.

Staffing structures for prevention work. SDVCs formed their staff-level prevention teams between 2002 and 2006, the period during which all DELTA Program SDVCs began receiving DELTA Program funding. One OPCQ item asked SDVCs to describe the purpose of their prevention team. The responses fell into two general categories: (1) to plan and coordinate prevention activities (e.g., training and technical assistance, especially those related to the DELTA Program); and (2) to build prevention capacity of the SDVC as an organization and of individual SDVC staff. During 2006, 7 of the 11 prevention teams met at least every two months; four met on a quarterly basis, with one of the teams that met on a quarterly basis reporting that part of the team also met on a monthly basis.

Operating structures for prevention capacity. In addition to establishing a prevention team, SDVCs reported having fully implemented other organizational structures that support planning, implementation, and evaluation of primary prevention activities (see Figure 2). For example, nine SDVCs included prevention activities in staff members' job descriptions, which is three-fourths of the 12 SDVCs

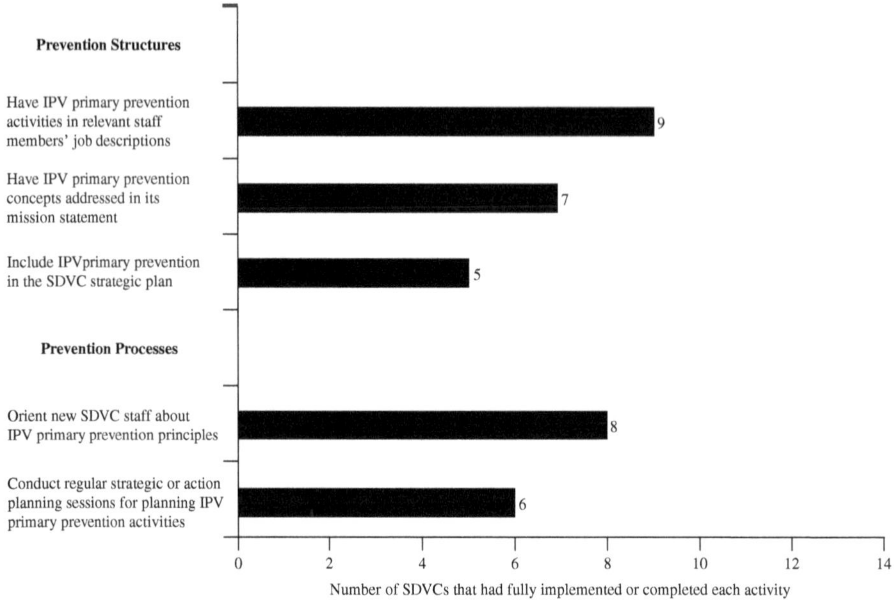

FIGURE 2 Primary Prevention Internal Capacity Building Activities Reported by DELTA SDVCs During 2006 (n = 14)

that reported having written job descriptions. Seven SDVCs reported that their mission statement addressed primary prevention concepts, which is more than half of the 12 SDVCs that reported having a written mission statement. Five SDVCs reported that they had included prevention in the SDVC strategic plan, which is more than half of the nine SDVCs that reported having a written strategic plan.

Resources. SDVCs reported on various resources that were intended to support their primary prevention activities. In terms of funding, the median percentage of the 14 DELTA SDVCs' annual budgets that was used for primary prevention was estimated at 15 per cent, ranging from 2 per cent to 37 per cent. DELTA Program awards in fiscal year 2006 ranged from $171,825 to $413,744, with the median award being approximately $190,000. The majority of each SDVC's award directly supported the primary prevention work of the 45 DELTA-funded CCRs. Outside of DELTA funds, for SDVCs the most common source of funding for primary prevention activities was state or local government (reported by 6 SDVCs), followed by federal funding, private foundation grants, and individual or corporate donations (5 SDVCs reported each of these sources).

SDVCs also reported on other resources available to their prevention teams for their prevention work. The 11 SDVCs reported their prevention teams had access to sufficient technological resources for communication, and nine indicated they had adequate meeting space, food, and materials for running meetings. Only three SDVCs reported their prevention teams had sufficient funding to travel to conferences and adequate access to data for planning; and two had sufficient access to professional development opportunities.

Organizational processes. In terms of organizational processes that support the SDVCs' prevention activities, 8 of the 14 DELTA SDVCs reported that they had fully implemented a process to orient new SDVC staff about IPV primary prevention principles, and six reported that they conducted regular strategic or action-planning sessions for planning IPV primary prevention activities (Figure 2). In open-ended questions, SDVCs reported other activities, such as holding a capacity-building retreat and ensuring that SDVC staff and board members were informed about DELTA work.

SDVC Primary Prevention Work. The DELTA Program SDVCs reported a variety of primary prevention activities that supported the work of prevention stakeholders receiving (i.e., the 45 DELTA-funded local CCRs) or not receiving DELTA funding. Examples of prevention stakeholders not receiving DELTA funding include: non-DELTA funded CCRs, government agencies (e.g., Children's Protective Services), colleges and universities, health care providers, the faith community, and elementary and secondary schools. All DELTA Program SDVCs reported providing primary prevention support – namely, training or technical assistance – to DELTA-funded CCRs and SDVC member organizations that serve victims of IPV and their children (see Figure 3). The least-frequently listed organizations to which SDVCs provided support were mental health and addiction programs and batterer programs.

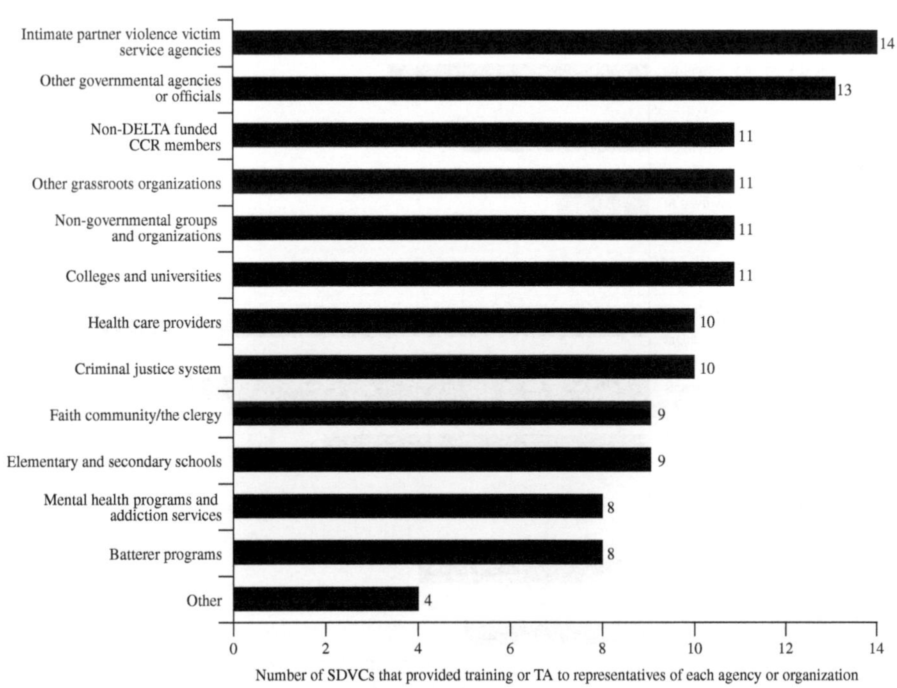

FIGURE 3 DELTA and non-DELTA IPV Prevention Stakeholders Receiving Prevention Support from DELTA SDVCs During 2006 (n = 14)

Prevention synthesis and translation activities. Seven of the 14 SDVCs reported they had fully incorporated IPV primary prevention concepts into local trainings (Figure 4). In addition, four SDVCs had completed development of an IPV curriculum around the principles of prevention (Nation et al., 2003), another six were in the process of developing such a curriculum, and three had not yet developed a curriculum. In open-ended questions, other synthesis and translation activities were reported by three SDVCs, including one that published a "Building Healthy Relationships" facilitator's guide and another that translated prevention materials from English into another language.

Prevention support activities. Ten SDVCs reported that they maintained primary prevention as a consistent element in conferences and regional trainings. Furthermore, to ensure quality and improvement with prevention support efforts, seven SDVCs used organized methods for evaluating SDVC training and technical assistance activities (see Figure 4). All SDVCs included community organizing; concepts of primary prevention; and public health themes, concepts, and practices in the content of their technical assistance and training efforts (see Figure 5). In addition, 13 SDVCs presented on such topics as evaluation planning, conducting needs assessments, and evidence-based planning; and 10 SDVCs conducted training on leadership development, group process and team building, and identifying evidence-based IPV primary prevention strategies.

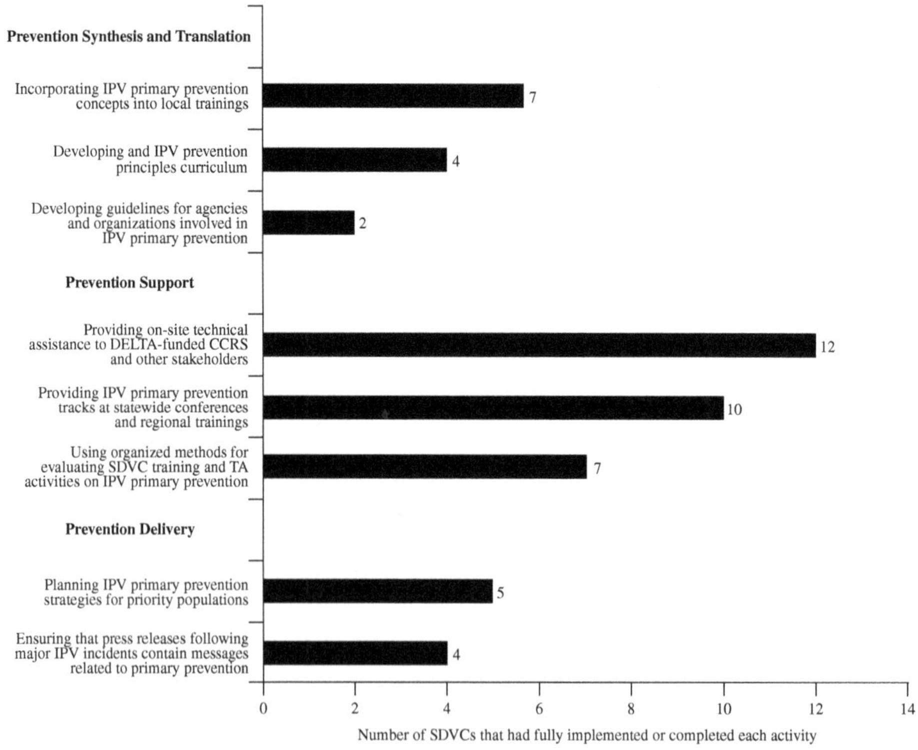

FIGURE 4 Primary Prevention Work Reported by DELTA SDVCs during 2006 (n = 14)

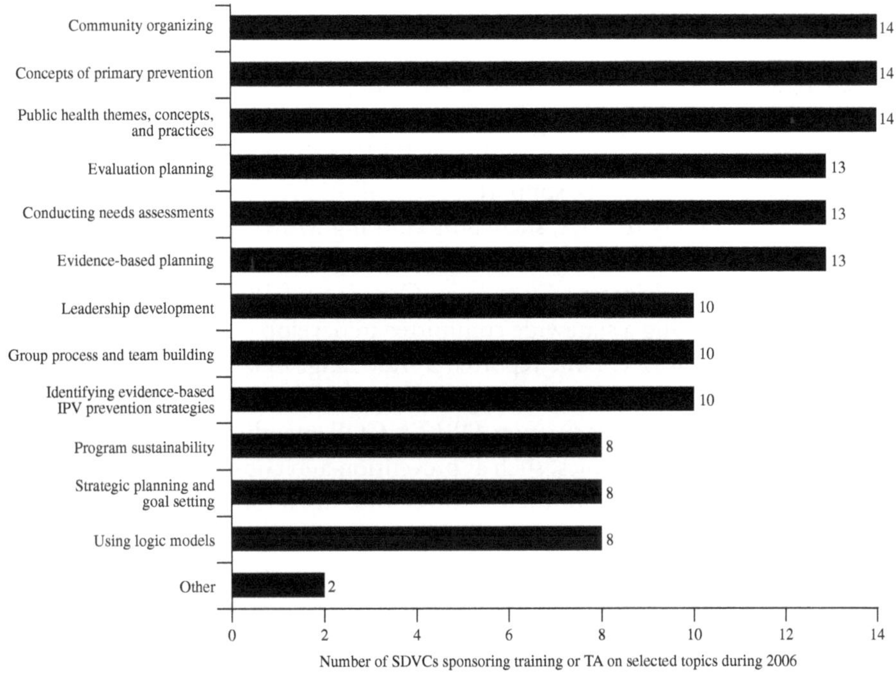

FIGURE 5 Content of Prevention Training and Technical Assistance Provided by DELTA SDVCs during 2006 (n = 14)

Prevention delivery activities. The DELTA SDVCs communicated primary prevention activities with DELTA funded and non-DELTA funded IPV prevention stakeholders through a variety of methods: workshops, seminars, and trainings (14 SDVCs); email or electronic mailing list ("listserv"; 14 SDVCs); statewide conferences (11 SDVCs); newsletters (10 SDVCs); written reports (8 SDVCs); and the SDVC website (8 SDVCs). Moreover, in open-ended questions, four SDVCs with a prevention team reported that they maintained or updated the SDVC website with materials developed through the DELTA Program.

Five SDVCs reported planning IPV primary prevention strategies for priority populations; two SDVCs reported such planning was in process. Four SDVCs worked to ensure that press releases following major IPV incidents contained messages related to primary prevention; two more reported that developing these messages was in process (see Figure 4). Other methods used to communicate with stakeholders were reported by five SDVCs in open-ended responses, including agency, program director, and state steering committee meetings; board trainings; site visits; press releases; and networking meetings.

Delivery activities supporting funded CCRs. When asked more specifically about their support of DELTA-funded CCRs, 13 SDVCs sponsored an event that CCR members attended and provided materials or resources to these CCRs; 12 SDVCs indicated their members attended one or more CCR-sponsored events. SDVCs also reported communicating regularly with the leadership or members of the DELTA-funded CCRs, with all SDVCs having in-person meetings with CCR leadership on at least a quarterly basis; 13 reported that they communicated by email on at least a weekly basis.

Delivery activities supporting non-funded CCRs. The DELTA SDVCs were asked to describe their interactions with non-DELTA funded CCRs. All 14 DELTA SDVCs provided prevention support to non-DELTA funded IPV prevention stakeholders in a variety of ways, such as by working with statewide stakeholders to increase IPV prevention components in their programming/funding criteria, providing national and international (e.g., Canada and Russia) trainings on IPV prevention, and forming a statewide committee to develop a state-level plan for the primary prevention of IPV. Nine reported a wide range of specific interactions and prevention support activities, such as providing training and technical assistance when requested, waiving fees for non-DELTA CCR members to attend trainings, providing information on topics, such as prevention and community organizing via electronic mailing lists and monthly mailings, offering a forum for DELTA CCRs to provide information to non-DELTA CCRs, inviting non-DELTA CCRs to attend state prevention conferences and regional workshops, and providing prevention strategic-planning technical assistance.

DISCUSSION

The assessment provides an overview of the 14 DELTA Program SDVCs' general capacity, primary prevention capacity, and primary prevention work during 2006. The findings provide information that could be used by practitioners to move primary prevention in the field from its formative stage to become more established. For example, no formalized models exist, nor did any emerge, of what are the most important elements of organizational capacity for pursuing IPV primary prevention. Instead, the findings illustrate an individualized approach to capacity building, as reflected by the variation in how the SDVCs leveraged current intervention support structures, involved SDVC leadership in their prevention work, developed their general and prevention capacity, and implemented prevention activities. In fact, each SDVC has been supported in its capacity building and prevention work in a manner that best suited its own organizational and state context and the needs of the DELTA funded CCRs. The findings suggest that for primary prevention of IPV, one size does not fit all.

SETTING THE STAGE FOR PRIMARY PREVENTION

As noted earlier, the CDC DELTA Program enabled DELTA SDVCs to complement the existing IPV intervention training and technical assistance infrastructures traditionally supported by SDVCs with primary prevention-focused training, technical assistance, and funding to local CCRs. It was not surprising, therefore, that the DELTA SDVCs successfully integrated primary prevention principles, concepts, and practices into the support activities for DELTA-funded CCRs. It was unexpected, however, the extent to which DELTA SDVCs were able to leverage their knowledge for other key stakeholders not receiving DELTA Program funding.

The DELTA Program used a variety of communication and collaboration methods to broaden the base of agencies and organizations that have a stake in preventing the occurrence of IPV. The DELTA Program SDVCs integrated primary prevention content into existing intervention-focused training and technical assistance infrastructures such as workshops, seminars, on-site trainings, statewide conferences and trainings, newsletters, regional trainings, email, and electronic mailing lists. Thus, SDVCs used a diverse set of approaches to leverage their existing intervention infrastructure and organizational networks to promote prevention, both within the DELTA-funded CCRs as well as within agencies and organizations that were not funded by the DELTA Program.

THE ROLE OF LEADERSHIP

In most cases, the SDVC executive director was a member of the prevention team, suggesting a high level of engagement and organizational buy-in for prevention capacity building and prevention work within the SDVC. The prevention teams are also a vehicle for executive directors to demonstrate their prevention leadership. However, the establishment of a prevention team with an executive director as an active member may not necessarily indicate that the SDVC formal leadership is actively engaged if the prevention team meets infrequently, such as every other month or quarterly. More needs to be known about the role that executive directors' play and how their formal leadership is "value-added," compared to a team comprised solely of SDVC staff. Future evaluation efforts might consider using qualitative methods to explore the roles, level of participation, and perceived impact of executive directors in building prevention capacity within the DELTA Program SDVCs.

THE LINK BETWEEN GENERAL AND PREVENTION CAPACITY

The assessment demonstrates the link between SDVCs' general capacity and prevention capacity. Research suggests that organizations with sufficient general capacity are able to more successfully implement new types of work and activities than organizations without sufficient general capacity (Livet, Courser, & Wandersman, 2008). The assessment findings expand on earlier research by indicating that the development of prevention capacity is associated with certain general capacity characteristics being established. As an example, although 12 SDVCs had a written mission statement, only six had a mission statement that incorporated primary prevention. These results indicate that institutionalizing, or building an organization's capacity for primary prevention requires attention not only to primary prevention content, but also to the development of more general structures and processes within the organization as a whole.

FUTURE EVALUATION ACTIVITY

This chapter has implications for the structure of future data collection and analysis related to SDVCs' prevention capacity building and prevention work. The DELTA Program evaluation resembles a "developmental evaluation" in which goals and outcomes evolve as learning takes place (Patton, 2008). The OPCQ was developed based on the best available science and practice knowledge regarding SDVC primary prevention capacity and primary prevention work at the time. While developed as a way to move effective programs, practices, and principles into the field, the ISF is a useful tool for understanding the interactions of the system components related to prevention synthesis and translation, support, and delivery. The ISF helped to retrospectively frame and enhance the work of the DELTA Program (Cox, Finklestein, Perez, & Rosenbach, 2010).

While the assessment sheds light on the prevention support activities of the DELTA SDVCs, less is known about their prevention synthesis and translation and delivery activities, in part because these roles have evolved over time, especially with the addition of empowerment evaluators to the DELTA team. The OPCQ contained limited questions on these activities for two main reasons. First, as primary prevention practice was still relatively new to all DELTA Program grantees, the knowledge and practice of primary prevention synthesis and translation activities was in its early development stage and is reflected as such in the data collection instrument. Second, the primary prevention synthesis and translation activities reported for the entire 2006 period probably do not reflect the work of the empowerment evaluators. The evaluators were not hired until late 2006 to assist SDVCs in synthesizing and translating DELTA Program prevention principles, concepts, and practices to meet each state's unique needs.

Similarly, the DELTA Program SDVCs reported few prevention delivery activities, again, because the OPCQ did not include many questions on prevention delivery activities given the limited knowledge and experience in the field at the time the survey was developed and conducted. Thus, a modified version of the OPCQ will be used in future evaluations to improve its ability to more accurately assess the developing practice of SDVC prevention synthesis and translation and prevention delivery activities.

LIMITATIONS

Several caveats affect the interpretation and generalizability of the findings from this chapter. First, the data were self-reported by the DELTA SDVCs and the measures regarding general capacity, prevention capacity, and prevention work have not been validated by an external source. Second, as this study includes only the 14 DELTA-funded SDVCS, these assessment results are not generalizable to SDVCs that have not been involved in the DELTA Program. Third, the results reported in this chapter reflect SDVC activities in 2006, one year into the three-year program period during which building organizational prevention capacity was a key focus; it is important to recognize that organizational change and capacity building take time. Thus, these results report the early steps these SDVCs took to build SDVC prevention capacity.

Finally, this chapter reports only cross-sectional data, and future evaluations would be beneficial for establishing a relationship between DELTA Program supports and increasing prevention capacity and prevention work. DELTA Program grantees reported prevention capacity, which is consistent with the primary prevention principles, concepts and practices promoted by CDC through the DELTA Program. With DELTA Program support, prevention teams were developed, and SDVCs expanded their reach beyond the usual IPV stakeholders.

CONCLUSION

This chapter documents the traditional and historical work of SDVCs, which has not been previously described in the literature despite 30 years of activity addressing IPV. The chapter also reports the results of an organizational prevention capacity questionnaire administered to DELTA Program SDVCs. Despite the limitations, the assessment results have already informed the work of the DELTA Program SDVCs and may expand beyond DELTA SDVCs to transform future activities of SDVCs not directly involved in the DELTA Program. Therefore, the seeds have been planted to move primary prevention of IPV from a formative stage into a more mature and naturally occurring practice. In time, the traditional work of SDVCs may come to include primary prevention alongside social change and intervention work.

ACKNOWLEDGEMENTS

The authors wish to express their sincere gratitude to the 14 DELTA State Domestic Violence Coalitions that graciously shared the data used in this chapter. The authors are also grateful to Janelle Moos (North Dakota Council on Abused Women's Services/Coalition Against Sexual Assault), Debby Tucker (National Center on Domestic and Sexual Violence), Allison Randall (Administration for Children and Families, U.S. Department of Health and Human Services), and Sandra Cashman (Centers for Disease Control and Prevention, U.S. Department of Health and Human Services) for reviewing early drafts of this chapter.

The findings and conclusions in this chapter are those of the authors and do not necessarily represent the official position of the Centers for Disease Control and Prevention. Also, the findings and conclusions do not necessarily represent the official position of Mathematica Policy Research.

REFERENCES

Centers for Disease Control and Prevention. (2006). *Understanding intimate partner violence fact sheet*. Retrieved May 1, 2009, from National Center for Disease Control and Prevention Web site: http://www.cdc.gov/ViolencePrevention/pdf/IPV-FactSheet.pdf.

Centers for Disease Control and Prevention. (2011). *Domestic Violence Prevention Enhancement and Leadership Through Alliances (DELTA)*. Retrieved April 3, 2012, from National Center for Disease Control and Prevention Web site: http://www.cdc.gov/ViolencePrevention/DELTA/index.html.

Cox, P. J., Finkelstein, D. M., Perez, V. E., Rosenback, M. L. (2010). Changes in capacity among local coordinated community response coalitions supported by the DELTA Program. *Journal of Family Social Work, 13* (4), 375-392.

Dahlberg, L. L., & Krug, E. G. (2002). Violence – a global health problem. In E. G. Krug, L. L. Dahlberg, J. A. Mercy, A. B. Zwi, & R. Lozano (Eds.), *World report on violence and health* (pp. 1-22). Geneva: World Health Organization.

Delaware Coalition Against Domestic Violence. (2004). *Overview and history*. Retrieved May 1, 2009, from http://www.dcadv.org/overview-and-history

Family Violence Prevention and Services Act. 42 U.S.C. §10410 (1994).

Family Violence Prevention and Services Act. 42 U.S.C. §10410 (1997).

Family Violence Prevention and Services Act. 42 U.S.C. §10418 (2002).

Family Violence Prevention and Services Act. 42 U.S.C. §10418 (2007).

Flaspohler, P., Duffy, J., Wandersman, A., Stillman, L., & Maras, M.A. (2008). Unpacking prevention capacity: An intersection of research-to-practice models and community-centered models. *American Journal of Community Psychology, 41*(3-4), 182-96.

Florida Coalition Against Domestic Violence. (n.d.). *Herstory*. Retrieved May 1, 2009, from http://www.fcadv.org/about

Johnson, M. P. (1995). Patriarchal terrorism and common couple violence: Two forms of violence against women in U.S. families. *Journal of Marriage and the Family, 57*, 283-294.

Livet, M., Courser, M., & Wandersman, A. (2008). The prevention delivery system: Organizational context and use of comprehensive programming frameworks. *American Journal of Community Psychology, 41*(3-4), 361-378.

Nation, M., Crusto, C., Wandersman, A., Kumpfer, K. L., Seybolt, D., Morrisey-Kane, E., & Davino, K. (2003). What works in prevention: Principles of effective prevention programs. *American Psychologist, 58*(6/7), 449–456.

National Network to End Domestic Violence [NNEDV]. (n.d.). *U.S. State and Territorial Coalitions*. Washington, D.C.: Author.

National Network to End Domestic Violence [NNEDV]. (2007). *Defining state domestic violence coalitions: Essential criteria*. Washington, D.C.: Author.

New York State Coalition Against Domestic Violence. (2008). *Herstory of the coalition.* Retrieved May 1, 2009, from http://www.nyscadv.org/herstory/

North Dakota Council on Abused Women's Services. (n.d.). *History*. Retrieved May 1, 2009, from http://www.ndcaws.org/about_us/history.html

Patton, M. Q. (2008.) *Utilization-Focused Evaluation*, 4th ed. Thousand Oaks, CA: Sage Publications, Inc.

Saltzman, L. E., Fanslow, J. L., McMahon, P. M., & Shelly, G. A. (1999). *Intimate partner violence surveillance: Uniform definitions and recommended data elements, Version 1.0.* Atlanta, GA: National Center for Injury Prevention and Control, Centers for Disease Control and Prevention.

Schechter, S. (1982). *Women and male violence: The visions and struggles of the battered women's movement.* Boston: South End Press.

U. S. Department of Health and Human Services, Administration on Children and Families [DHHS-ACF]. (1995). 60 Fed. Reg. 9033 (February 16, 1995).

U. S. DHHS-ACF. (1997). 62 Fed. Reg. 4055 (January 28, 1997).

U. S. DHHS-ACF. (2001). 66 Fed. Reg. 63139 (December 4, 2001).

U. S. DHHS-ACF. (2003). 68 Fed. Reg. 18232 (April 15, 2003).

U. S. DHHS-ACF. (2004). 69 Fed. Reg. 5167 (February 3, 2004).

U. S. DHHS-ACF. (2005). 70 Fed. Reg. 31483 (June 1, 2005).

U.S. DHHS-ACF. (n.d.). FY 2009 FVPSA Grant Announcements: Background Information. Washington, D. C.: Author.

U. S. Department of Health and Human Services, Centers for Disease Control and Prevention [DHHS-CDC]. (2002). Domestic Violence Prevention Enhancement and Leadership Through Alliances (DELTA) Program, 67 Fed. Reg. 49696 (July 31, 2002).

U. S. DHHS-CDC. (2005). Domestic Violence Prevention Enhancement and Leadership Through Alliances (DELTA) Program, 70 Fed. Reg. 9320 (February 25, 2005).

U. S. Department of Justice, Office on Violence Against Women [DOJ-OVW]. (2009). Grants to state sexual assault and domestic violence coalitions program. Retrieved February 10, 2009, from U.S. Department of Justice Web site: http://www.ovw.usdoj.gov/ovwgrantprograms.htm#16

Wandersman, A., Duffy, J., Flaspohler, P, Noonan, R., Lubell, K., Stillman, L, Blachman, M., Dunville, R., & Saul, J. (2008). Bridging the gap between prevention research and practice: The interactive systems framework for dissemination and implementation. *American Journal of Community Psychology, 41*(3-4), 171-181.

The Rape Prevention and Education (RPE) Theory Model of Community Change: Connecting Individual and Social Change

PAMELA J. COX and KAREN S. LANG
Centers for Disease Control and Prevention, Atlanta, Georgia

STEPHANIE M. TOWNSEND
Consultant, Pittsford, New York

REBECCA CAMPBELL
Department of Psychology, Michigan State University, East Lansing, Michigan

Social work practice has long focused on the connections between an individual and the social environment that affect the individual's social functioning. The Rape Prevention and Education (RPE) Program's theory model, Creating Safer Communities: The Rape Prevention and Education Model of Community Change, provides family social workers with a framework for examining and changing the individual and social factors that lead to sexual violence. This model connects two societal change theories, community readiness and diffusion of innovations, with three individual level theories, theory of reasoned action, theory of planned behavior and the health belief model, for the purpose of ending sexual violence. The Centers for Disease Control and Prevention (CDC) created this theory model to promote the use of theory-based prevention strategies among RPE Program grantees. In this article the authors (1) describe the theoretical underpinnings of the RPE theory model; (2) explore how one RPE grantee, supported with funding from the EMPOWER Program, used the RPE theory model to create a state sexual violence prevention plan; and (3) discuss how family social workers can utilize the model to promote sexual violence prevention within their own states and communities.

As noted by Cox, Ortega, Cook-Craig, and Conway (this issue), sexual violence (SV) is a significant problem that affects millions of individuals and families as well as society as a whole. Social workers have long been involved in addressing SV at individual and societal levels by providing crisis intervention and counseling services to sexual assault survivors, advocating for appropriate SV prevention and intervention policies, and mobilizing communities to confront and prevent SV (Stout & McPhail, 1998). With a heightened awareness that SV is preventable, social workers can extend the scope of their efforts to end SV by applying the Rape Prevention and Education (RPE) Program's theory model, Creating Safer Communities: the Rape Prevention and Education Model of Community Change, to their individual and social change work.

The RPE Program was established at the Centers for Disease Control and Prevention (CDC) by the 1994 Violence Against Women Act. The purpose of the RPE Program is to strengthen sexual prevention efforts in all 50 states, the District of Columbia, Puerto Rico, and six U.S. territories. The RPE Program contains a mixture of individual and social-level change elements. Individual educational seminars (for professionals, the public, and schools, colleges and universities); the operation of crisis hotlines; and the development of informational materials on such topics as how to reduce one's risk of victimization or where to receive services. Since 2005, social change elements have included promoting social norms that reduce the risk of SV, state- and community-level strategic planning, community mobilization, coalition building, and policy reform.

CDC modified the RPE Program in 2005 to include a mixture of individual and social change elements, which reflect social work's person in environment approach (National Association of Social Workers [NASW], 2005). Prior to this modification, an assessment of the RPE Program by CDC (Clinton-Sherrod et al., 2004) and the research literature indicated that the SV prevention field had limited capacity to implement and evaluate individual-level strategies that had a reasonable chance to prevent SV, due to the structure of the strategies. No primary prevention social change strategies could be identified among state and community organizations supported by RPE funds or in the research literature. Specific structural challenges with the individual level strategies were (1) a lack sufficient dosage (e.g., a one-time 45-minute presentation) (Nation et al., 2003); (2) content that addressed myths about sexual assault and provided information on legal definitions of SV, signs of potential perpetrators, and local resources for victims (e.g., Lenihan, Rawlins, Eberly, Buckley, & Masters, 1992; Pinzone-Glover, Gidycz, & Jacobs, 1998) but provided few skill-building opportunities for participants; (3) audiences of mixed genders; and (4) the lack of a theoretical base.

Across health areas, research suggested that, for individual-level strategies to have a reasonable chance to prevent the problem health behavior (e.g., SV perpetration), participants must receive a sufficient dosage (i.e., multiple sessions) of the content and opportunities to build the skills that prevent the problem behavior (Nation et al., 2003). Although attitude change may be necessary to change behavior, it is not sufficient nor is it long lasting. In the case of SV prevention, research indicated that individual-level SV prevention strategies were able to reduce rape-supportive attitudes (e.g., Fonow, Richardson, & Wemmerus, 1992; Heppner, Good, et al., 1995; Holcomb, Sarvella, Sondag, & Holcomb, 1993; Lenihan & Rawlins, 1994; Mahlstedt, Falcone, & Rice-Spring, 1993; Shultz, Scherman, & Marshall, 2000), but that the gains in attitude change diminished over time (e.g., Heppner, Humphrey, Hillenbrand-Gunn, & Debord, 1995). Additionally, research on SV strategies suggested that single-gender audiences experienced higher attitudinal change than mixed-gender audiences (Brecklin & Forde, 2001). In sum, in the early 2000s, there was strong practice and research evidence that the standard individual-level practices of rape prevention organizations, low dosage, didactic presentations to mixed-gender audiences that focused on knowledge and attitude change, were insufficient to achieve the type of sustained behavioral change that would prevent first-time perpetration (Gidycz et al., 2001).

The specific framework that CDC's Division of Violence Prevention uses in its RPE Program to understand the person in the environment is the social ecological model, which posits that there is a complex interplay of individual, relationship, community, and societal factors that contribute to the occurrence of SV. Through this model, state and community organizations supported by RPE funds are able to address the underlying multidimensional, multilevel causes of SV (Nation et al., 2003) rather than simply focus on changing individuals. Today, CDC works with state and community organizations supported by RPE funds to develop, implement, and evaluate SV primary prevention strategies at all levels of the social ecology.

As noted above, one key structural issue with RPE Program individual-level strategies was the lack of an identified theoretical base that could explain how behavior change was intended to occur. This issue, along with the fact that no societal-level SV primary prevention strategies could be identified, led CDC to develop a theory of change model for the RPE Program that encompassed both individual and societal level change. The Creating Safer Communities: Rape Prevention and Education Model of Community Change (RPE theory model) was developed with input from state and community organizations supported by RPE funds and other stakeholders. The RPE theory model provides these organizations and other audiences with an understanding of the types of strategies needed to pursue multilevel change and articulates how change happens at the community and individual levels. Family social workers can utilize this model to inform their efforts to seek individual, family, and society-level changes in their communities and states. This article explains the theoretical underpinnings of the RPE theory model and how to apply this model for ending SV by exploring how one RPE grantee used the model to guide stakeholders in their development of a state SV prevention plan. The article closes by discussing specific implications for family social work practice.

THEORETICAL FOUNDATION OF THE RPE THEORY MODEL

The RPE theory model is based on community-level theories, community readiness and diffusion of innovation (DOI), and individual-level theories, theory of reasoned action (TRA), theory of planned behavior (TPD), and the health belief model (HBM). These theories, along with their implications for SV prevention, are discussed in this section.

Community Readiness Theory

Like many other social problems with multilevel causes, SV prevention efforts require involvement from broad sectors of the community. However, different sectors within a community may be at different levels of readiness to engage in SV prevention. Some sectors or individuals in the community may be aware that SV is a local problem, whereas other sectors and individuals may deny or minimize its existence in the community. Finally, there may be another entire segment of the local community that may be aware of the problem but has little understanding of what can be done to address it. Without sufficient readiness, prevention strategies often fail (Edwards, Jumper-Thurman, Plested, Oetting, & Swanson, 2000).

The theory of community readiness is a helpful tool to assess the readiness of various groups and the community as a whole to address a particular program and to identify the types of efforts that are appropriate to address the problem given the community's state of readiness (Plested, Smithman, Jumper-Thurman, Oetting, & Edwards, 1999). Originally developed and tested in the area of substance abuse prevention, the theory provides a framework for understanding community processes and outlines the stages communities go through as readiness increases (Edwards et al., 2000; Plested et al., 1999). The model assesses communities along six dimensions and assigns the community to one of nine stages of readiness: (1) existing community efforts such as programs, activities, and policies; (2) community knowledge of the efforts; (3) leadership, including appointed leaders and influential community members; (4) community climate; (5) community knowledge about the problem; and (6) resources for prevention such as people, money, time, and space (Edwards et al., 2000; Plested et al., 1999). The nine resulting stages are (1) no awareness: the issue is not recognized by the community or its leaders as a problem; (2) denial: the community feels that the problem does not exist or that nothing needs to be done about it; (3) vague awareness: the problem is recognized, but there is no motivation for acting. Ideas about why the problem occurs tend to be vague or rely on stereotypes. No identifiable leadership exists or leadership lacks motivation for doing anything about the problem; (4) preplanning: the problem is recognized, and there is common agreement that something needs to be done. There are identifiable leaders, but efforts are not focused; discussion is happening but no real planning to address the problem is under way; (5) preparation: leadership is active, and planning is under way with decisions about tasks and responsibilities being made and resources being sought; (6) initiation: an activity or action is under way but is viewed as a new effort; (7) stabilization: one or two strategies are operating and are expected to continue for the foreseeable future; however there is no evaluation of effectiveness and tracking of prevalence may or may not be occurring; (8) confirmation/expansion: the limitations of the existing strategies are recognized, and attempts are under way to improve them. Resources are being sought or committed for new, expanded efforts; and (9) professionalization: prevention efforts are marked by sophistication, training, and effective evaluation (Edwards et al., 2000; Plested et al., 1999).

Individually, family social workers can only do so much to promote societal-level change. With broad support, SV prevention efforts can succeed. By conducting a readiness assessment, family social workers and their partners can identify the stage of readiness of key organizations and segments of the community and develop activities to increase the organizations' readiness to engage in societal-level change efforts focused at SV prevention. As a community's level readiness for SV prevention increases, family social workers and their partners can use DOI and individual change theories to plan, develop, and implement and evaluate specific prevention strategies.

Diffusion of Innovation

Rogers' (1995) DOI theory explains how an innovation, such as a SV prevention practice, can be spread throughout the community to saturate the community with new ideas or principles; this saturation leads to the emergence of new community norms. For the RPE Program and SV prevention, DOI theory requires saturating communities with ideas, information, and skills (i.e., innovations) that lead to the prevention of SV and the promotion of positive social norms and behaviors such as safety, equality, and respect. A critical element of DOI theory is that changing community norms will lead to changes in individuals' behavior. For many practitioners in the anti-SV field, this is a new orientation to SV prevention, as most efforts to date have focused on individual change, based on the belief that if enough individuals change their attitudes and behavior, then community change will result. For family social workers, this orientation is not necessarily new, due to their work with systems theory and the social work focus on person in environment; however, the application of the DOI to such work may be new.

DOI theory was selected as a theoretical foundation of the RPE theory model because it is conceptually consistent with the social-ecological model and has been empirically tested using community-level interventions for HIV prevention and found to be a sound approach (Kegeles, Hay, & Coates, 1996; Kelly, St. Lawrence, Brasfield, Lemke, et al., 1990; Kelly, St. Lawrence, Brasfield, Stevenson, et al., 1990; Kelly et al., 1991; Miller, Kotz, & Eckholdt, 1998; Sommerville, Diaz, Davis, Coleman, & Taveras, 2006). Although HIV prevention attempts to change different behaviors and norms than SV prevention, both issues require multilevel change, both address issues of stigma and discrimination, and both exist within an environment characterized by social pressure to keep quiet. DOI theory has yet to be tested in the specific context of SV prevention. In fact, there are no studies in the published scientific literature that provide empirical support for any community change model for SV prevention.

In brief, DOI theory has four main elements: innovation, communication, time, and social systems (Rogers, 1995). *Innovation* refers to "an idea, practice, or object that is perceived as new by an individual or other unit of adoption" (Rogers, 1995, p. 11). The key point is that it is perceived as new. Even developing a positive attitude toward something that one previously had a negative attitude toward would qualify as a perceived new idea. The second element is the communication channels (e.g., mass media or interpersonal contact) by which the innovation is spread from one person or unit to another (Rogers, 1995). The third element is time. Time considers the process by which an innovation is adopted and how quickly it is adopted (Rogers, 1995). The last element is the social system through which an innovation is diffused.

Two key aspects of DOI theory that have particular implications for SV prevention practice are communication channels and the social system through which the innovation is diffused. The element of communication channels has important implications for the types of strategies communities employ. Communication channels include interpersonal, face-to-face exchanges of information and mass media.

Interpersonal channels, which focus on individual-level change, are seen as more effective than mass media in persuading people to adopt a new behavior; however, the persuasion is even more effective when the people involved in the interpersonal communication are similar (Rogers, 1995). This issue of similarity is a key one for RPE Program grantees and family social workers as they are unlikely to be persuasive with people who are unlike them. Most SV prevention strategies target youth and young adults, and more and more strategies are focusing on young males to prevent first-time perpetration of SV. For these strategies to be effective, the people who deliver them need to be similar to the people receiving them. Specifically, they need to be relatively young and male. Thus, RPE Program grantees and family social workers may be more effective in their SV prevention efforts by partnering with community organizations that have staff that are similar to the SV prevention target audiences and have expertise in working with these audiences. Another option is for RPE Program grantees and family social workers to recruit and train volunteer opinion leaders, who are similar personally and professionally with the target audiences, to deliver prevention messages.

Mass media is often appealing as a communication channel through which to promote social change due to its ability to broad reach. However, this broad reach does not lead to behavior change as effectively as face-to-face communication (Rogers, 1995). Additionally, mass media is resource intensive and may exert influence in a small segment of the population who are exposed to a great deal of mass media, have large social networks, seek out information, and worry less about the consequences of the innovation (Rogers, 1995). Consequently, limited prevention resources may be best used on face-to-face communication channels utilizing various partners in a variety of settings.

In addition to communication channels, the social networks where the innovation or strategy is introduced have implications for SV prevention (Rogers, 1995). Social networks may be the people and institutions within a community, service area, or a priority population that span multiple settings. The structure of the social network, in particular the norms, change agents, and opinion leaders, can affect the introduction and adoption of an innovation (Glanz, Rimmer, & Lewis, 2002). As the most innovative change agent within a social network may be seen as too radical, these change agents may not be as influential as someone who is more integrated into the mainstream (Glanz et al., 2002). To the extent that sexual assault crisis agency staff and family social workers are seen as radical change agents within their own communities, they should consider partnering with mainstream opinion leaders to introduce and sustain the SV prevention messages or strategies. The development of such partnerships may be a key outcome of utilizing community readiness theory introduced earlier.

Finally, it is important to consider the tendency of those promoting an innovation to focus on increasing awareness, which often means awareness the innovation exists (e.g., SV prevention) (Glanz et al., 2002), not necessarily knowledge on how to adopt the innovation. However, how-to knowledge is the most important consideration in whether someone decides to adopt the innovation. Therefore, strategies like bystander intervention, which build individuals' skills to recognize unhealthy or problematic behavior and intervene in an appropriate manner (e.g., confronting sexist language), incorporate a how-to component that is critical to the actual adoption of a commitment to SV prevention and subsequent changes in societal, institutional, family, and individual behaviors (Banyard, Moynihan, & Plante, 2007).

Individual Behavior Change Theories

Sexual violence occurs within social contexts that vary in the degree to which such behaviors are condoned or promoted. However, most individuals living within any given social context do not commit SV. Therefore, prevention strategies must address social norms and individual behaviors. Changing community norms through strategies based on DOI theory should provide the necessary conditions to promote individual behavior change. Yet, to create actual individual behavior change, the RPE theory model draws upon three specific individual behavior change models: TRA, TPB, and the HBM. The National Institute of Mental Health identified the points of consensus among the theories: (1) the individual has positive intention to perform the behavior, (2) there are no environmental constraints against performing the behavior, and (3) the individual has the skills to perform the behavior (Fishbein et al., 1991). Fishbein et al. (1991) also identified five factors that influence the strength of the intention to perform the behavior: (1) the benefits of having a positive attitude toward the behavior outweigh the costs, (2) the individual perceives more social pressure to perform the behavior than to not perform it, (3) the individual views the behavior as consistent with his or her self-image, (4) the individual believes he or she has the capability to perform the behavior, and (5) the individual's emotional reaction to the behavior is positive (Fishbein et al., 1991). Empirical evidence from the health promotion area of changing sexual practices supports the theories of individual behavior change (Albarracin, Johnson, Fishbein, & Muellerleile, 2001; Crepaz & Marks, 2002; Koniak-Griffen & Stein, 2006; Posner, Bull, Ortiz, & Evans, 2004; Serovich & Greene, 1997). In considering application of these theories to other health behaviors, it has been argued that, to change behavior, it is important to have reinforcement or aversive consequences in place (Biglan, 1995). Reinforcement involves social approval for performing the behavior one wishes to promote and taking away the benefits of the behavior one wishes to prevent (Biglan, 1995).

In thinking specifically about SV prevention, applying the theories of individual behavior change gives rise to a number of considerations for state and community organizations supported by RPE funds and family social workers. First, severe negative consequences need to be associated with committing acts of SV. Because an attitude toward a behavior can be influenced by something associated with it, associating SV with severe negative social consequences (e.g., prosecution, social ostracism, effects on daily life, etc.) could make the attitude toward committing SV more negative. Most state and community organizations supported by RPE funds and family social workers have been at the forefront of advocating for such negative consequences for more than three decades and their work at creating an environment intolerant of SV should continue. Second, social norms must be changed so that there is pressure not to engage in SV and pressure to engage behaviors that promote safety, equality, and respect. Additionally, the physical and social environment must constrain SV-related behaviors and promote behaviors that lead to safety, equality, and respect. This may involve bystander intervention training in which individuals increase their sense of efficacy in intervening in high-risk situations or in or addressing comments and norms that contribute to a rape-supportive culture.

USING THE RPE THEORY MODEL TO GUIDE STATE-LEVEL SV PREVENTION PLANNING

The RPE theory model was created to inform state and community organizations supported by RPE funds' development of theory-based prevention strategies and to strengthen prevention efforts throughout communities. To put the theory model into practice while building capacity for planning and evaluation among state and community organizations supported by RPE funds, CDC created the EMPOWER (Enhancing and Making Programs and Outcomes Work to End Rape) Program. In 2005 the CDC awarded 3-year cooperative agreements to a subset of states supported by RPE funds: Colorado, Massachusetts, North Dakota, and North Carolina. Kentucky and New Jersey joined EMPOWER but received no operating funds. The key task of EMPOWER Program participants was to develop a state-level prevention plan in an inclusive manner. Thus, each EMPOWER participant convened a state prevention team that had authentic representation from the diverse communities within their states. To promote capacity building, all EMPOWER states worked with an external evaluator who followed the principles of empowerment evaluation set forth by Fetterman and Wandersman (2004). All EMPOWER states used the RPE theory model to guide their planning efforts.

An illustrative case study of New Jersey's EMPOWER Program is presented to show how the RPE theory model has influenced the development of one state's SV prevention plan and how the successes and challenges in using the RPE theory model to guide programmatic decision making reflected DOI theory. This illustrative case study involved in-depth interviews conducted with the EMPOWER coordinator and empowerment evaluator. New Jersey was selected for the case study based on the high degree of expertise and experience using the RPE theory model to guide planning efforts as demonstrated by the training and technical assistance the New Jersey team has provided at national RPE grantee meetings. The case study provides family social workers with an example of how the RPE theory model can be used to help partners understand and act upon key primary prevention concepts.

The New Jersey EMPOWER Program and its state plan-development process was spearheaded by a state capacity-building team made up of staff from the Department of Community Affairs, Division on Women; the Department of Health; and the New Jersey Coalition Against Sexual Assault; and an empowerment evaluator. State capacity-building teams, a requirement of the EMPOWER program, are designed to support the broader state prevention team. The New Jersey state capacity-building team developed a prevention team composed of 35 members representing state government agencies and state and community nonprofit organizations, to develop the New Jersey SV prevention plan. This prevention team expanded of the Governor's Council against SV, Prevention and Public Education Committee.

The state capacity-building team increased the capacity of the state prevention team to conduct a data-driven planning process informed by the RPE theory model. Thus, the capacity-building team facilitated the planning process and introduced the RPE theory model and its application in developing a plan for preventing SV. The empowerment evaluator had the unique role of being a coach to the capacity-building and prevention teams in how to use data and the RPE theory model, develop and prioritize goals, and identify strategies to achieve goals as part of the overall planning process.

Reflecting DOI theory, the state capacity-building team used the RPE theory model as a tool to introduce several innovations in preventing SV to the prevention team: perpetration prevention, societal and systems change focus, and community readiness. Recognizing that potential victims should not and cannot be responsible for preventing their own victimization, all of the states in CDC's EMPOWER Program focus on preventing perpetration, rather than victimization. Having the prevention team embrace a perpetration prevention focus, however, was not an easy task for two structural reasons. First, the SV prevention field has historically focused on preventing victimization by increasing women's knowledge about rape and how to reduce their risk of victimization. Second, as the data related to the magnitude of SV are mostly victimization data, prevention team members had a tendency to focus on how to reduce the victimization rates right in front of them rather than how to reduce the unknown, and undocumented, perpetration rates. However, the RPE theory model's articulation of long-term outcomes focused on the prevention of SV perpetration and the promotion of safety, equality, and respect helped the prevention team embrace a perpetration prevention focus.

In New Jersey, like the rest of the country, most SV prevention efforts focused on individual change, not societal or systems change. The state capacity-building team wanted the prevention team to consider strategies at multiple levels of the social ecology. Given the dominant focus on individual-level strategies and the relative lack of community and societal level change strategies for SV prevention, the state capacity-building team anticipated that a focus on societal and systems change would present a challenge for the prevention team. Thus, the RPE theory model was used to (1) explore potential societal and systems level strategies and (2) shift the frame from implementing individual-level change strategies with the hope these individual strategies would bring about community change *to* implementing community-level change strategies that might eventually bring about individual change.

The state capacity-building team introduced the RPE theory model to the prevention team in the early stages of conducting the needs and resources assessment. After the initial introduction, the model was distributed at two other key junctures in the planning process. The first key juncture was at the start of developing goal and outcome statements, to keep the prevention team focused on preventing perpetration and promoting positive social norms. The second key juncture was when identifying strategies to keep the prevention team focused on all levels of the social ecological model. To help guide strategy selection, the capacity-building team reinforced the concepts in the RPE theory model by sharing another tool, a literature review that described the theories and related research that supported the RPE theory model.

The adoption and use of the theories and concepts in the RPE theory model by prevention team members reflected DOI theory. The minority of prevention team members who had a background in research immediately understood the importance and direction offered by the RPE theory model and its embedded theories (e.g., community readiness, TRA). These prevention team members were the early adopters who quickly integrated the model's key concepts of perpetration prevention, societal and systems change focus, and community readiness into their planning efforts. The literature review helped other members understand and use the model and its related theories in their planning efforts. Through formal and informal leadership roles, the early adopters were instrumental in helping the entire prevention team to embrace a focus on preventing perpetration, consider societal and system change strategies, and take into account community readiness (i.e., diffusing the innovation) when planning for SV prevention.

Formal roles of the early adopters included chairing or cochairing subgroups of the planning team devoted to specific tasks in the planning process. For example, one of the early adopters cochaired a subgroup charged with identifying strategies for one of the goals in the state plan. The subgroup was making progress on identifying system change strategies until the cochair went on leave. Because there had not been enough time for the focus on perpetration prevention and system change strategies to become the norm, the subgroup reverted back to focusing on preventing victimization through individual change strategies. When the cochair returned, the subgroup regained its focus on preventing perpetration through systems change strategies. This example reflects the element of

DOI theory that face-to-face information exchange can be more persuasive than other information channels (in this case, written information that was provided by the capacity-building team).

Informally, other prevention team members would look to the early adopters for direction and input. Although the capacity-building team encouraged the leadership of the early adopters, their informal leadership roles came about organically as the early adopters became more engaged in the planning process due to their better understanding of how to apply the concepts within the RPE theory model. This greater engagement resulted in the early adopters wanting to take on more leadership roles and speaking up in meetings more often than they had previously. Reflecting DOI theory in action, the early adopters may have been seen as credible messengers regarding the utility of the RPE theory model to the planning process due to other prevention team members viewing the early adopters as more similar themselves than the capacity-building team members. As the capacity-building team was in charge of facilitating the planning process and introducing the RPE theory model and its use in developing a plan for preventing SV, thus prevention team members may have viewed the capacity-building team members as authority figures, rather than peers, and dissimilar to themselves.

Although many of the prevention team members reported that they did not fully understand the RPE theory model and all of its underlying theories, all prevention team members eventually came to support and endorse the focus on preventing perpetration through strategies at all levels of the social ecology and participated fully in the process to identify and select strategies.

Looking retrospectively, the New Jersey EMPOWER coordinator reflected that having more concrete examples of strategies, whether focused on SV prevention or other health issues, that are based on the various theories that make up the theory model, would have made the concepts more accessible more quickly to all prevention team members, not just those with backgrounds or interest in theory and research. Providing such examples was beyond the ability of the capacity-building team due to the limited timeframe and the resources available to complete the state-level SV prevention plan.

CONCLUSION

The RPE theory model and the New Jersey example of its application to state-level SV prevention planning provide family social workers with theoretical guidance and practical knowledge on how to apply social work's person in environment principle to SV prevention. As the person in environment principle means that a person can only be understood within the environment within which that person lives, the RPE theory model provides an understanding of how individual change and community change are linked, and it suggests how to design prevention strategies to reach the intended audience and have an impact. An effective SV prevention must address the underlying causes of SV and be based on validated theories of behavior and/or social change (Nation et al., 2003), the RPE theory model is built on the theories of community readiness (Plested et al., 1999) and diffusion of innovation (Rogers, 1995) as well as multiple individual behavior change theories (Fishbein et al., 1991). The key premise of this model is that there must be sustained effort to saturate communities with messages and expectations that are intolerant of SV and promote positive social norms such as safety, equality, and respect to change community-level norms. Efforts to change community-level norms can then reinforce individual behavior change. Multiple theories of individual behavior change emphasize that people need reinforcement to change their behaviors.

Although the concept of saturation and widespread introduction of information often invoke the idea of mass media communication, DOI theory and its supporting empirical evidence suggest that having key opinion leaders directly engaged with their community constituents can be more effective. Because key opinion leaders are "local" to the community and are highly regarded and respected, the weight of their message is particularly impactful. Mass media campaigns may be best used in SV prevention to reinforce messages that are simultaneously being communicated through more interpersonal communication channels.

The New Jersey case example provides a practical application of the entire RPE theory model and DOI theory, in particular. For family social workers wanting to promote SV prevention, this case example suggests that they need to build broad-based partnerships to tap the key opinion leaders from multiple sectors within their communities. Based on New Jersey's experiences, social workers who use the RPE theory model to guide planning and other SV prevention efforts should be prepared to (1) continually revisit the model at multiple points with their partners, (2) encourage the leadership of early adopters, and (3) have concrete examples of strategies from SV prevention or other fields that are based on the theories in the model. Following the RPE theory model and lessons learned from the New Jersey case example, family social workers can work with key partners to identify, develop and/or adapt, and implement prevention strategies that have a greater likelihood of preventing the initial perpetration of SV and achieving positive social change.

ACKNOWLEDGEMENTS

CDC would like to acknowledge the work of Dr. Rebecca Campbell and Dr. Stephanie Townsend in conducting the literature review and developing the RPE theory model. The authors express their gratitude to all of the state and community organizations supported by RPE funds and stakeholders who reviewed and provided comment on the various iterations of the RPE theory model. They also wish to express their sincere gratitude to the New Jersey EMPOWER Team, who so graciously shared their experiences in utilizing the RPE theory model in their state-planning efforts.

REFERENCES

Albarracin, D., Johnson, B. T., Fishbein, M., & Muellerleile, P. A. (2001). Theories of reasoned action and planned behavior as models of condom use: A meta-analysis. *Psychological Bulletin, 127*, 142–161.

Banyard, V. L., Moynihan, M. M., & Plante, E. G. (2007). Sexual violence prevention through bystander education: An experimental evaluation. *Journal of Community Psychology, 35*, 463–481.

Biglan, A. (1995). *Changing cultural practices: A contextualist framework for intervention research*. Reno, NV: Context Press.

Brecklin, L. R., & Forde, D. R. (2001). A meta-analysis of rape education programs. *Violence and Victims, 16*(3), 303–321.

Clinton-Sherrod, M., Spencer, D., Morrison, S., Lenfestey, N., Fornnarino, L., & Kuo, T. (2004). *Evaluability assessment of the rape prevention and education program*. Unpublished report (Contract No. 200-2001-00123). Research Triangle Inc., NC.

Cox, P. J., Ortega, S., Cook-Craig, P., & Conway, P. (2010). Strengthening systems for the primary prevention of sexual violence and intimate partner violence: CDC's EMPOWER and DELTA programs. *Journal of Family Social Work, 13*(4), 287–296.

Crepaz, N., & Marks, G. (2002). Towards an understanding of sexual risk behavior in people living with HIV: A review of social, psychological, and medical findings. *AIDS, 16*, 135–149.

Edwards, R. W., Jumper-Thurman, P., Plested, B. A., Oetting, E. R., & Swanson, L. (2000). Community readiness: Research to practice. *Journal of Community Psychology, 28*(3), 291–307.

Fetterman, D. M., & Wandersman, A. (Eds.). (2004). *Empowerment evaluation principles in practice*. New York: Guilford Press.

Fishbein, M., Bandura, A., Triandis, H. C., Kanfer, F. H., Becker, M. H., & Middlestadt, S. E. (1991). *Factors influencing behavior and behavior change* [Final report of the NIMH theorist's workshop]. Washington, DC: National Institute of Mental Health.

Fonow, M. M., Richardson, L., & Wemmerus, V. A. (1992). Feminist rape education: Does it work? *Gender and Society, 6*, 108–121.

Gidycz, C. A., Layman, J. M., Rich, C. L., Crothers, M., Bylys, J., Matorin, A., & Jacobs, C. D. (2001). An evaluation of an acquaintance rape prevention program: Impact on attitudes, sexual aggression, and sexual victimization. *Journal of Interpersonal Violence, 16*, 1120–1138.

Glanz, K., Rimer, B. K., & Lewis, F. M. (2002). *Health behavior and health education: Theory, research, and practice*. San Francisco: Jossey Bass.

Heppner, M. J., Good, G. E., Hillenbrand-Gunn, T. L., Hawkins, A. K., Hacquard, L. L., Nichols, R. K., et al. (1995). Examining sex differences in altering attitudes about rape: A test of the elaboration likelihood model. *Journal of Counseling and Development, 73*, 640–647.

Heppner, M. J., Humphrey, C. F., Hillenbrand-Gunn, T. L., & DeBord, K. A. (1995). The differential effects of rape prevention programming on attitudes, behavior, and knowledge. *Journal of Counseling Psychology, 42*, 508–518.

Holcomb, D. R., Sarvela, P. D., Sondag, K. A., & Holcomb, L. C. H. (1993). An evaluation of a mixed-gender date rape prevention workshop. *Journal of American College Health, 41*, 159–164.

Kegeles, S. M., Hays, R. B., & Coates, T. J. (1996). The Mpowerment project: A community level HIV prevention intervention for young gay men. *American Journal of Public Health, 86*, 1129–1136.

Kelly, J. A., St. Lawrence, J. S., Brasfield, T. L., Lemke, A., Amidei, T., & Roffman, R. E. (1990). Psychological factors that predict AIDS high-risk versus AIDS precautionary behavior. *Journal of Consulting and Clinical Psychology, 58*, 117–120.

Kelly, J. A., St. Lawrence, J. S., Brasfield, T. L., Stevenson, L. Y., Diaz, Y. E., & Hath, A. C. (1990). AIDS risk behavior patterns among gay men in small southern cities. *American Journal of Public Health, 80*, 416–418.

Kelly, J. A., St. Lawrence, J. S., Diaz, Y. E., Stevenson, L. Y., Hauth, A. C., Brasfield, T. L., et al. (1991). HIV risk behavior reduction following intervention with key opinion leaders of population: An experimental analysis. *American Journal of Public Health, 81*, 168–171.

Koniak-Griffin, D., & Stein, J. A. (2006). Predictors of sexual risk behaviors among adolescent mothers in a human immunodeficiency virus prevention program. *Journal of Adolescent Health, 38*, 297.e1–297.e11.

Lenihan, G. O., & Rawlins, M. E. (1994). Rape supportive attitudes among Greek students before and after a date rape prevention program. *Journal of College Student Development, 35*, 450–455.

Lenihan, G. O., Rawlins, M. E., Eberly, C. G., Buckley, B., & Masters, B. (1992). Gender differences in rape supportive attitudes before and after a date rape education intervention. *Journal of College Student Development, 33*, 331–338.

Mahlstedt, D., Falcone, D. J., & Rice-Spring, L. (1993). Dating violence education: What do students learn? *Journal of Human Justice, 4*, 101–117.

Miller, R. L., Klotz, D., & Eckholdt, H. M. (1998). HIV prevention with male prostitutes and patrons of hustler bars: Replication of an HIV intervention. *American Journal of Community Psychology, 26*, 97–131.

Nation, N., Crusto, C., Wandersman, A., Kumpfer, K. L., Seybolt, D., Morrissey-Kane, E., et al. (2003). What works in prevention: Principles of effective prevention programs. *American Psychologist, 58*(6/7), 449–456.

National Association of Social Workers. (2005). *NASW standards for clinical social work in social work practices*. Washington, DC: Author.

Pinzone-Glover, H. A., Gidycz, C. A., & Jacobs, C. D. (1998). An acquaintance rape prevention program: Effects on attitudes toward women, rape-related attitudes, and perceptions of rape scenarios. *Psychology of Women Quarterly, 22,* 605–621.

Plested, B. A., Smithman, D. M., Jumper-Thurman, P., Oetting, E. R., & Edwards, R. W. (1999). Readiness for drug abuse prevention in rural minority communities. *Substance Use & Misuse, 34,* 521–544.

Posner, S. F., Bull, S. S., Ortiz, C., & Evans, T. (2004). Factors associated with condom-use among young Denver inner-city women. *Preventive Medicine: An International Journal Devoted to Practice and Theory, 39,* 1227–1233.

Rogers, E. M. (1995). *Diffusion of innovations* (4th ed.). New York: Free Press.

Serovich, J. M., & Greene, K. (1997). Predictors of adolescent sexual risk-taking behaviors which put them at risk for contracting HIV. *Journal of Youth and Adolescence, 26,* 429–444.

Shultz, S. K., Scherman, A., & Marshall, L. J. (2000). Evaluation of a university-based rape prevention program: Effect on attitudes and behavior related to rape. *Journal of College Student Development, 41,* 193–201.

Somerville, G. G., Diaz, S., Davis, S., Coleman, K. D., & Taveras, S. (2006). Adapting the popular opinion leader intervention for Latino young migrant men who have sex with men. *AIDS Education and Prevention, 18A,* 137–148.

Stout, K. D., & McPhail, B. (1998). *Confronting sexism and violence against women: A challenge for social work.* New York: Longman.

Using Social Network Theory to Influence the Development of State and Local Primary Prevention Capacity-Building Teams

PATRICIA G. COOK-CRAIG

School of Social Work, University of Kentucky, Lexington, Kentucky

This article examines the role that social network theory and social network analysis has played in assessing and developing effective primary prevention networks across a southeastern state. In 2004 the state began an effort to develop a strategic plan for the primary prevention of violence working with local communities across the state. The process included an analysis of how family service organizations and community collaborators networked to solve community problems. In 2005, the state joined the Center for Disease Control and Prevention's Enhancing and Making Programs Work to End Rape project to specifically focus on building capacity for primary prevention of perpetration of sexual violence.

This article presents an examination of how assumptions of social network theory were used to design a strategy for the assessment of professional networks and the development of a state prevention team and local community networks committed to primary prevention of sexual violence. Social network theory and analysis examines the connections between people or entities. A quantitative analysis of survey data on networks of professionals working in agencies committed to violence prevention was conducted as part of a needs assessment and state profile of violence in a southeastern state. Social network analysis techniques were used to examine how 139 community partners across 10 local regions in the state collaborated with one another. The social network analysis findings were used to design strategies for building a state prevention team and engaging in capacity-building activities at the state and local level to ensure a successful process of developing a primary prevention plan for the perpetration of sexual violence. First, the article begins a brief description of the structure of the violence prevention planning process in the state. Then a literature review that defines the assumptions behind social network theory that are salient to the primary prevention planning process is outlined. A review of how social network theory intersects with the effectiveness of coalitions is provided. The article then reviews findings examining the state's regional violence prevention provider networks. Finally implications for building violence prevention planning teams, engaging in family social work, and conducting further research in this area are considered.

BACKGROUND: PLANNING FOR PRIMARY PREVENTION OF PERPETRATION OF SEXUAL VIOLENCE

In 2004, the state began an effort to develop a strategic plan for the primary prevention of violence working at the state and local levels. One of the goals was to develop well-functioning coalitions in regions across the state. These coalitions were tasked with the development of statewide and regional capacity to enhance primary prevention of violence (see Cook, Morris, & Kelly, 2006). As part of this effort, regional teams participated in an analysis of how family service organizations and community collaborators networked together to solve community problems. That same state joined the Enhancing and Making Programs Work to End Rape (EMPOWER) project in 2005 to specifically focus on building statewide capacity for primary prevention of perpetration of sexual violence (for a detailed description of the EMPOWER program, see Cox, Ortega, Cook-Craig, & Conway, 2010/this issue). The organization of activities for the EMPOWER project was guided by a small planning team called the State Capacity Building Team (SCBT). The initial activity of the state's EMPOWER project was to convene a state prevention team (SPT) tasked with developing a statewide primary prevention plan specifically designed to address perpetration of sexual assault. This plan was developed using a planning process called Getting To Outcomes (GTO) (for a detailed description of the GTO framework, see Cox et al., 2010/this issue). The same network analysis data that was collected as part of the strategic planning process was then used to inform the work of the SPT. To demonstrate how that data was used in the planning process, it is necessary to first review basic assumptions behind social network theory.

Social Network Theory and Analysis

Social network theory describes the set of assumptions that underlies how actors (including individuals and entities such as organizations) connect with one another. Two assumptions of social network theory that are particularly important in understanding how community partnerships are formed are related to the concepts *homophily* and *propinquity*. *Homophily* refers to the assumption that, other factors being the same, individuals and entities are likely to connect to others with whom they share similar characteristics. *Propinquity* refers to the assumption that other factors being constant, individuals and entities are likely to connect with those that are geographically close to them (Kadushin, 2004).

Social network analysis is the process by which researchers explain the nature of relations in a network and how that might affect outcomes. An underlying assumption of social network analysis is that individuals or entities in a network are interdependent members and that resources flow through those relationships. The process of conducting social network analysis involves examining the structure of networks and looking for patterns that explain how networks facilitate or constrain resource exchange (Galaskiewicz & Wasserman, 1994).

Visualization techniques allow for the examination of the structure of social networks. By creating representations of network members and their connections with one another, patterns in networks can be identified and communicated (Knoke & Yang, 2008). The process of creating social network maps first appeared in the social work literature in the early 1990s as a tool for understanding the social support networks of client (see Tracy, 1993; Tracy & Abell, 1994). More recently it has been used how community agencies connect with one another (Orthner, Cole, & Erhlich, 2000).

The Connections Between Community Collaborations and Social Network Theory

Research on evaluating community coalitions suggests that these types of collaborations struggle with the success they have at involving a broad array of constituencies and at meeting their stated objectives (Kadushin, Lindholm, Ryan, Brodsky, & Saxe, 2005). Lack of success in these areas can be related to the difficulties associated with getting the needed people to the table and working effectively together. Networks are naturally inclined to include homophilous relations, in which members have similar experiences, backgrounds, and professional philosophies (see Kadushin, 2004), and collaboration can be difficult when the group comprises diverse constituencies with different perspectives (Kadushin et al., 2005). However, it is just the diverse set of resources and ideas inherent in a heterogeneous coalition made up of constituencies from different disciplines, agencies, and backgrounds that is necessary to engage in solving complex problems (Wolff, 2001). This necessitates engaging nontraditional partners as coalition members.

Even though the research on community coalitions has shown mixed success in meeting state goals and including diverse partners at the table, many scholars continue to recognize the importance of collective action in communities and have turned their attention to uncovering strategies that will increase the likelihood of working groups and coalitions success (Foster-Fishman, Berkowitz, Lounsbury, Jacobson, & Allen, 2001; Koslowski, & Ilgen, 2006; Wolff, 2001). Wolff (2001) highlighted the importance of a diverse, inclusive membership as necessary for a successful coalition; in network terms this means that a key aspect of building successful coalitions is to actively resist the natural inclination to build a homophilous team. In addition, Koslowski and Ilgen (2006) demonstrated the importance of leadership and how prominent team members work to create effective teams and guide effective collaborative action.

Social Network Theory and the Applicability to Community Collaborations Building

The social network theory concepts of strong versus weak ties is also a useful way of understanding how the network of community partners that work together can make a difference in the success of community collaborations. Community collaborations offer key stakeholders access to new connections of professionals they are not currently connected to, which can be called weak ties. Granovetter (1973, 1982) introduced the concept of strong versus weak ties between individuals, which suggests that there are two different types of connections that offer different benefits. According to Granovetter (1973), strong ties are relational bonds that exist between "similar people." These relationships involve relationships between people with similar characteristics and provide a connection to a common identity, shared purpose, trust, and an efficient source of information and resource sharing (Burt, 2001; Putnam, 2000; Warren, Thompson, & Saegart, 2001; Woolcock & Narayan, 2000).

On the other hand, weak ties connect people who have heterogeneous characteristics (Burt, 2001; Putnam, 2000; Woolcock & Narayan, 2000; Warren et al., 2001). Granovetter (1973) hypothesized that weak ties provide new opportunities for individuals to be introduced to a broader range of resources. Weak ties are facilitated through common connections, such as friends of friends, who can introduce one another. Because new relationships are formed, new opportunities to share information and resources are created.

The concept of weak and strong ties can be applied to professional relationships as well (see Hansen, 1999; Haythornthwaithe & Wellman, 1998; Krackhardt, 1992). Among professional networks, *strong ties* refer to relationships between workers that have regular contact with one another. Weak ties exist between professionals who do not have regular contact. Weak ties offer the opportunity to gain new knowledge and ways of practice across organizations and disciplines. They are important to community collaborations because the problems addressed by these collaborations are complex and need multidisciplinary solutions and widespread buy-in to put new solutions to work on the ground.

Engaging weak ties is also an important factor in addressing community readiness to engage in primary prevention of violence. Two important dimensions of community readiness to make change are community knowledge of the issue and community knowledge of the efforts to address the issue (Plested, Edwards, & Jumper-Thurman, 2006). By engaging a broad base of community partners from different disciplines, organizations, and backgrounds, practitioners can increase the likelihood that needed knowledge of the issue and the change effort will reach the larger community.

Because weak ties can be important to successful community collaboration, a network assessment of the types of collaborative relationships that communities rely on when conducting prevention planning can be useful in determining the extent to which needed heterogeneous partners are at the table. The discussion that follows outlines one state's efforts to engage in such an assessment.

METHOD

To better understand the ways in which regional providers work together, a social network analysis (SNA) was conducted to determine how organizations connect with one another on a regular basis. SNA is an analytic strategy used to examine the nature of the relations between people in various types of networks (in this case, their regional service provider networks) (Wasserman & Faust, 1994). SNA is particularly useful to establish trends and patterns of how organizations collaborate or network together.

Sample

As a facet of the statewide effort to create a violence prevention plan, the SCBT engaged regional partners from across the state to complete a social network assessment designed to explore how regional family service organizations, prevention programs, and other community collaborators connect with one another. In each region of the state, a team of practitioners and community stakeholders interested in violence prevention had been formed. A snowball sampling technique was used to identify key stakeholders who would be potential respondents and who were considered key collaborative partners in the community. Snowball sampling techniques have been found to be a useful technique to identifying social network membership which can be hard to identify in cases (Frank, 2005) such as uncovering community collaborators. For this project, the analysis was based on a sample of 139 service providers and community collaborators that represented 10 regions of the state.

Instrument Development

To assess how community partners networked to collaborate on behalf of their clients, a 10-item asset assessment questionnaire was developed that captured information on referral patterns from people in agencies, organizations, or groups that work with victims and perpetrators of violence. Respondents were also asked to provide a bounded list of the top five agencies that they referred to and received referrals from.

This strategy was designed to be a preliminary analysis of how regions are networked and begins to provide a picture of the differences in how regions work together. The bounded nature of the asset assessment questionnaire allowed for an analysis of the most salient relationships that providers had with other agencies and stakeholders in the community; however, it could not represent the entire network of providers in any one of the regions.

Data Analysis

The data were input into an SPSS (Version 15) data file for analysis. In addition, the data were used to employ network visualization techniques to determine the structure of the networks in each region to search for patterns or trends across regions. Once this work was completed, findings were reported back to each region, as a form of member checks. Respondents were able to provide comments on how accurate the network type identified for their region reflected collaborative work on a regular basis.

FINDINGS

Common Collaborative Relationships

Respondents reported a variety of organizational types with whom they shared working relationships. In total, 60 different types of organizations and community groups were named as frequent collaborative partners. Of these 60 types, 40% were nontraditional violence prevention partners. *Nontraditional violence prevention partners* were defined as those partners who can play a needed role in helping to prevent violence but that have not worked in the field of violence or actively participate in violence prevention planning or activities. Collaborators were considered nontraditional if their mission or programs did not include regular work with victims or perpetrators of violence. Examples of nontraditional partners included housing programs, community mental health providers, private doctors, and businesses. This suggests that practitioners in the region were connecting to nontraditional partners, engaging weak ties is instrumental in developing new information and resources needed to move forward in the violence prevention planning process.

The most common collaborative partner in the regions was the local community mental health center. This is an important finding in relationship to community violence prevention planning in light of local policies. Due to safety concerns, local community mental health centers in the state do not provide services to known perpetrators of violence. This makes them an unlikely partner in primary prevention of perpetration of violence; however, primary prevention collaborators name them as the organization that they most often depend on as a referral source.

Other common sources of collaboration included child welfare, domestic violence programs, rape crisis centers, hospitals, law enforcement (such as the police and the courts), faith-based programs, schools, health departments, and private physicians.

Types of Community Networks

Network visualization techniques were used to identify a typology of network structures in the 10 regions. It was clear from the analysis that the way regions network and collaborate together varies from location to location. In fact, service providers who work with victims and perpetrators of violence from different regions across the state had different network patterns. In exploring the data on the relationships of networks of violence providers across regions in the state, three main "types" of network structures emerged that explain how organizations connect with one another.

Each network "type" has a different style of using its organizational and relational resources to meet the needs of their communities. Any successful violence prevention effort must recognize these different ways of working together and how regional networks work (or fail to work) together to solve problems. Because the regional challenges are different, technical assistance and support around building optimal networks that can facilitate violence prevention should be tailored to the type of network involved in change.

Type 1: Loosely connected networks

Two of the 10 regions had loosely connected networks (see Figure 1). In these networks, the groups of organizations/providers that work on problems associated with violence tend to work largely independently and provide and receive referrals from a unique set of organizations/providers. The network relies on one agency that tends to be the agency that all network members connect through. Although this creates an imbalance in how agencies are linked together, it does provide a clear picture as to how to begin connecting organization and clients together. When thinking of planning primary prevention activities, technical assistance around building

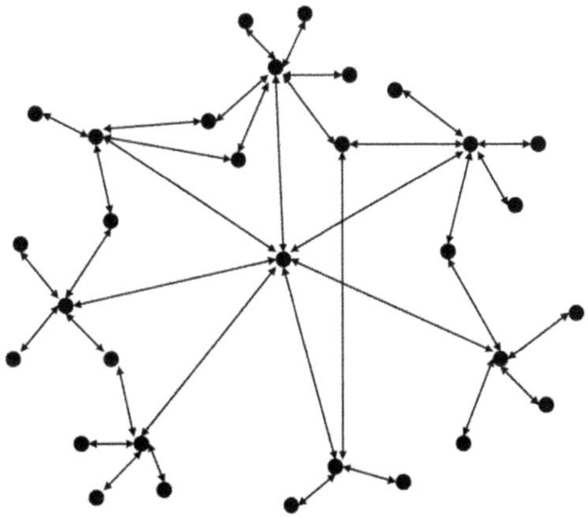

FIGURE 1 Loosely connected network.

optimal network structures would be an important component of working in these regions. This entails beginning by building relationships between potential partners through the use of weak ties. Time in planning meeting must be spent on increasing the strength of members' relationships prior to asking them to work on tasks related to prevention planning.

TYPE 2: NETWORKS LINKED BY HUBS

Four regions had networks that operated around "hubs" (see Figure 2). In networks linked by hubs, organizations tend to connect to a small set of organizations/providers that act as hubs to connect the broader set of groups that work together. These hubs can be centralized around an organization type or a geographic area. When thinking of planning primary prevention activities, these hubs can be a natural selection for a beginning point to connect people and organizations to the roll out of primary prevention activities.

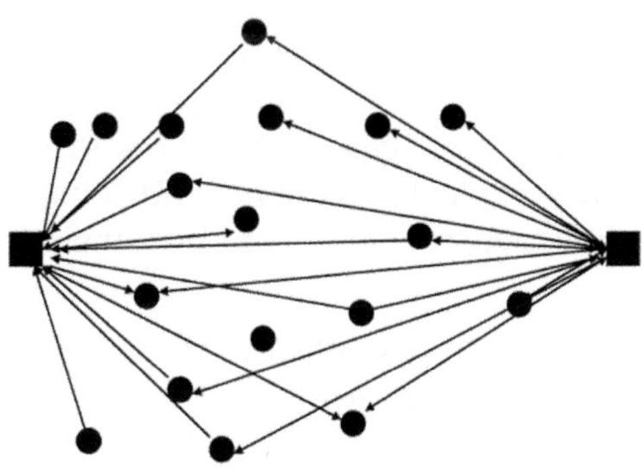

FIGURE 2 Hub network.

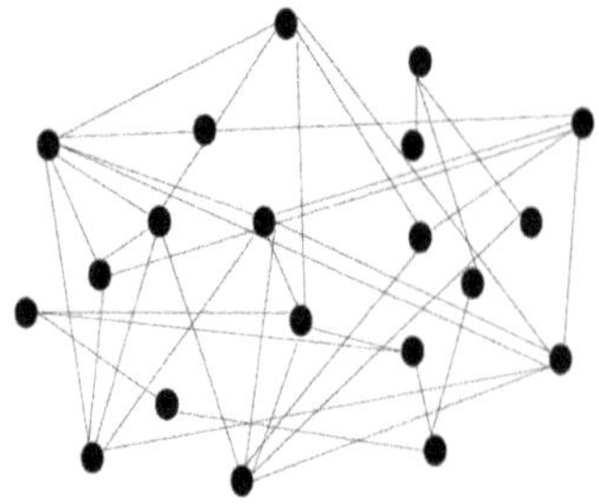

FIGURE 3 Fully-connected network.

TYPE 3: FULLY CONNECTED NETWORKS

Four regions had networks whose members were highly integrated with each other (see Figure 3). In these regions, organizations reported many connections to one another. The network of providers working together is not dependent on a small subset of organizations that seem to link other organizations together. These regions are not in need of technical assistance to assist in building integrated relationships because organizations already seem to be integrated. When thinking of planning primary prevention activities, these regions would need to consider how to disperse prevention activities across the entire set of organizations.

DISCUSSION

Using Social Network Theory to Assess Community Collaborations

Social network theory provided a framework in the state prevention planning project that is the focus of this article for clarifying the contextual factors that contribute to the ways in which professionals connect with one another and to help the regional planning groups to examine the design and membership of their workgroups and coalitions. Preliminary examination of these professional regional networks across the state focused on engaging in understanding how regions built their prevention networks and the role that homophily, or like characteristics, played in network development. This examination showed that violence prevention providers and advocates in regions across the state networked together differently. In fact, three "types" of network structures were identified among 10 regions in the state. A number of nontraditional partners were invited to the table and were invested in violence prevention work (Cook et al., 2006).

Applying the Findings to the Development of State Sexual Violence Primary Prevention Team

Having completed the network assessment, SCBT members shifted their focus to using the findings for two main purposes. First, the team used this strategy and the findings to build a state prevention team whose charge would be to develop a prevention plan of sexual violence perpetration. The network analysis data allowed SCBT members to profile the types of traditional and nontraditional partners that were already engaged in violence prevention planning and could be tapped to work on the issue of primary prevention of the perpetration of sexual violence. It also allowed for analysis of who has not been at the prevention planning table that varied from region to region. In their member checks, some regions reported that the visual interpretation of the network "type" was accurate; others expressed surprise that specific partners were not reflected in the picture. By using network assessment strategies and visualization techniques, it provided an avenue for important discussions of who the members that the group assumed would be at the table. In addition it provided concrete information that could be used to ensure that missing stakeholders could be recruited to join the group. This also opened discussion on the roles that people play in the planning process.

Second, the SCBT members used this data and this experience to plan and execute training and technical assistance to community members to build their own community teams who will serve to implement prevention strategies in their own communities. As the state developed its primary prevention plan and began to plan for implementation they recognized the importance of providing training and technical assistance on assessing collaborative partners, community readiness (particularly around the issue of knowledge and connection to the issue), the importance of the inclusion of nontraditional partners, and the need for a heterogeneous group of collaborative partners with a diverse set of knowledge and skills that can be tapped to build a successful change effort. By recognizing that communities collaborate differently, the SCBT was prepared to develop training tailored to helping local communities work within their own community to develop collaborative community teams that reflect the unique nature of the community, thereby increasing the likelihood that the team will work effectively.

Limitations of the Assessment Findings

The network data that were collected cannot be considered representative of the entire network of collaborative partners in each community. Because respondents were asked to name a bounded set of network relations, they only named the strongest collaborative relationships. Additional collaborative relationships do exist but were not captured due to the selected methodology for collecting network data. Conversely, there were also instances in which members were able to name the top five relationships in each question, but they could only name fewer than five.

In addition, the findings presented in the current study are not generalizable to all programs or communities. The purpose of conducting the network analysis was to assist the state and the participating communities to identify and strengthen their partnerships. Other communities would need to replicate the study methodology to understand who their collaborative partners are and to describe the nature and configuration of their partnership networks.

CONCLUSION

Community change processes are difficult and require multidimensional solutions with broad-based support (Wolfe, 2001). Historically the process of developing planning teams has been to invite anyone who was interested and invested to "come to the table." However, as shown earlier in this article, research on community change efforts suggests that this has not been effective. The infusion of social network theory into the development of community collaborations allows members strategies for engaging in deliberate decision making around who to invite to the table. This new way of assessing coalition and collaborative work can be successful at helping family service organizations become more efficient and effective at engaging community collaborations to prevent violence.

This has direct implications for how family social workers engage with other practitioners, providers, and stakeholders in the community. The findings and theoretical orientation that frames the current study suggest that family social workers can play a new role in prevention planning and coalition work. The assessment skills that social workers are trained to master should be put to work to explore, assess, and strengthen their own work groups. This can then be the beginning of a stronger coalition who will work more effectively on behalf of families and communities.

The science of how to engage community members to be a part of violence prevention work is young. Much more research is needed however on the impact of how communities network together to solve complex problems. Specifically, research on how different types of collaborative networks affect violence prevention outcomes is needed. By demonstrating that communities across a state operate with different network structures, this article is a first step in making the case that this research is needed. This requires a greater commitment by community coalitions and planning groups to evaluate whether their activities are successful in meeting the goals of the group. When coalitions are not successful in meeting their goals one possible explanation to explore is whether the members effectively network together or whether all the key players to make the initiative successful are participating.

REFERENCES

Burt, R. S. (2001). Structural holes versus network closure as social capital. In N. Lin, K. S. Cook, & R. S. Burt (Eds.), *Social capital theory and research* (pp. 31–56). New Brunswick, NJ: Transaction Publishers.

Cook, P. G., Morris, F., & Kelly, N. (2006). *Kentucky statewide violence prevention strategic plan*. Frankfort, KY: Cabinet for Health and Families.

Cox, P. J., Ortega, S., Cook-Craig, P., & Conway, P. (2010). Strengthening systems for the primary prevention of sexual violence and intimate partner violence: CDC's DELTA and EMPOWER programs. *Journal of Family Social Work, 13*(4), 287–296.

Foster-Fishman, P. G., Berkowitz, S. L., Lounsbury, D. W., Jacobson, S., & Allen, N. A. (2001). Building collaborative capacity in community coalitions: A review and integrative framework. *American Journal of Community Psychology, 29*, 241–261.

Frank, O. (2005). Network sampling and model fitting. In P. J. Carrington, J. Scott, & S. Wasserman (Eds.), *Models and methods in social network analysis* (pp. 31–56). Cambridge, UK: Cambridge University Press.

Galaskiewicz, J., & Wasserman, S. (1994). Introduction: Advances in the social behavioral sciences from social network analysis. In S. Wasserman & J. Galaskiewicz (Eds.), *Advances in social network analysis: Research in the social and behavioral sciences* (pp. xi–xvii). Thousand Oaks, CA: Sage.

Granovetter, M. (1973). The strength of weak ties. *American Journal of Sociology, 78*, 1360–1380.

Granovetter, M. (1982). The strength of weak ties: A network theory revisited. *Sociological Theory, 1*, 201–233.

Hansen, M. T. (1999). The search-transfer problem: The role of weak ties in sharing knowledge across organizational subunits. *Administrative Science Quarterly, 44*, 82–111.

Haythornthwaite, C., & Wellman, B. (1998). Work, friendship, and media use for information exchange in a networked organization. *Journal of the American Society for Information Science, 49*, 1101–1114.

Kadushin, C. (2004). Some basic network concepts and propositions. In *Introduction to social network theory*. Retrieved from http://stat.gamma.rug.nl/snijders/Kadushin_Concepts.pdf

Kadushin, C., Lindholm, M., Ryan, D., Brodsky, A., & Saxe, L. (2005). Why is it so difficult to form effective community coalitions? *City & Community, 4*, 255–275.

Knoke, D., & Yang, S. (2008). *Social network analysis* (2nd ed.). Thousand Oaks, CA: Sage.

Koslowski, S. W. J., & Ilgen, D. R. (2006). Enhancing the effectiveness of work groups and teams. *Psychological Sciences in the Public Interest, 7*(3), 77–124.

Krackhardt, D. (1992). The strength of strong ties: The importance of philos in organizations. Networks and organizations: Structure, form, and action. In N. Nohria & R. Eccles (Eds.), *Networks and organizations: Structure, form, and action* (pp. 216–239). Boston: Harvard Business School Press.

Orthner, D. K., Cole, G., & Erhlich, R. (2000). *Smart Start Collaboration network analysis report*. Chapel Hill: University of North Carolina Jordan Institute for Families. Retrieved from http://www.fpg.unc.edu/~smartstart/Reports/Smart-Start-June-2000-report.pdf

Plested, B. A., Edwards, R. W., & Jumper-Thurman, P. (2006). *Community readiness: A handbook for successful change*. Fort Collins, CO: Tri-Ethnic Center for Prevention Research.

Putnam, R. D. (2000). *Bowling alone: The collapse and revival of American community*. New York: Simon & Schuster.

Tracy, E. M. (1993). Teaching about social work and social support: A social network mapping exercise. *Journal of Teaching in Social Work, 7*, 37–46.

Tracy, E. M., & Abell, N. (1994). Social network map: Some further refinements on administration. *Social Work Research, 18*, 56–60.

Warren, M. R., Thompson, J. P., & Saegart, S. (2001). The role of social capital in combating poverty. In M. R. Warren, J. P. Thompson, & S. Saegart (Eds.), *Social capital and poor communities* (pp. 1–28). New York: Russell Sage Foundation.

Wasserman, S., & Faust, K. (1994). *Social network analysis: Methods and applications*. Cambridge, UK: Cambridge University Press.

Wolff, T. (2001). A practitioner's guide to successful coalitions. *American Journal of Community Psychology, 29*, 173–191.

Woolcock, M., & Narayan, D. (2000). Social capital: Implication for development theory, research, and policy. *World Bank Research Observer, 15*, 225–249.

Building the Capacity of States to Ensure Inclusion of Rural Communities in State and Local Primary Violence Prevention Planning

PATRICIA G. COOK-CRAIG
School of Social Work, University of Kentucky, Lexington, Kentucky

KAREN G. LANE
Montana Coalition Against Domestic and Sexual Violence, Helena, Montana

WENDI L. SIEBOLD
Evaluation, Management & Training Associates, Seattle, Washington

Rural, frontier, and geographically isolated communities face unique challenges associated with ensuring that they are equal partners in capacity-building and prevention planning processes at the state and local level despite barriers that can inhibit participation. By their nature, rural, frontier, and geographically isolated communities and states experience geographical isolation from planning partners and differential funding and staffing for prevention programming, as compared to urban or metropolitan states and local communities. At the same time, rural populations can face heightened risk associated with intimate partner violence (IPV) and sexual violence (SV) that intensifies the need to promote an inclusive primary prevention planning process that allows equal access of remote stakeholders to decision making related to prevention programming. This article presents a case study of two states to examine challenges and innovative solutions associated with ensuring inclusivity of rural and frontier communities in the Enhancing and Making Programs Work to End Rape and Domestic Violence Prevention Enhancements and Leadership Through Alliances violence prevention programs. Challenges associated with inclusion of rural communities in the planning process are presented, such as difficulty associated with participation due to geographic isolation. Innovative solutions, such as the use of technology designed to decrease these barriers that were used to bring together practitioners and state planners in these communities, are also presented. In addition, difficulties in ensuring that strategies are relevant to local culture are discussed.

Rural communities face unique challenges associated with ensuring inclusiveness in capacity-building and prevention planning processes for local planning groups and in state-level planning teams. States that are designated as rural or frontier have unique issues related to how to engage their communities in prevention planning. By their nature, rural, frontier, and geographically isolated communities experience geographical isolation from planning partners and differential funding and staffing for prevention programming as compared to urban or metropolitan communities. Family service agencies and their staff needing to participate in the planning process face challenges that can seem insurmountable and may opt out of participating. The result is that their voices in the process are marginalized. At the same time, rural populations may face heightened risk associated with intimate partner violence (IPV) and sexual violence (SV) that intensifies the need to promote inclusivity in primary prevention planning.

The purpose of this article is to present a case study of two states' efforts to increase inclusiveness regarding rural, frontier, and geographically isolated communities in their state and local planning processes to prevent SV and IPV. The two states, Kentucky and Montana, were participating in Centers for Disease Control and Prevention (CDC) funded projects (called Domestic Violence Prevention Enhancements and Leadership Through Alliances [DELTA] and Enhancing and Making Programs Work to End Rape [EMPOWER]) designed to build the capacity of state and local communities to engage in strategies aimed at primary prevention of perpetration of SV and IPV. The article begins by presenting a brief description of the planning process. Next rural, frontier, and geographically isolated communities are defined to provide a foundation for understanding the types of states that are profiled in the case study. An overview of the intersection between rurality and risk of violence is presented. The article then describes the case study methodology used in the current study and provides descriptions of the two programs included in the case study. Specific attention is paid to the empowerment evaluation principle of inclusion and its importance in prevention planning work in rural and frontier states and their local communities. A presentation of the challenges, opportunities, and innovative solutions associated with ensuring inclusivity of rural communities in the EMPOWER and DELTA violence prevention planning programs follows.

Finally the article highlights how rural capacity-building work is critical to and can enhance the work of family social work professionals in the field of violence prevention and intervention.

A NEW WAY OF APPROACHING PRIMARY PREVENTION PLANNING: THE CDC EMPOWER AND DELTA PROJECTS

In 2002, the CDC initiated a move toward helping states to build capacity to engage in primary prevention of perpetration of IPV and SV. Two outgrowths of the shift in focus were the DELTA and EMPOWER Programs. The focus of these two projects is to provide training and technical assistance to states to build capacity and create a plan for the primary prevention of perpetration of IPV and SV. The goal of this planning was to help states and local communities create a prevention plan to select new strategies designed to promote the prevention of perpetration of violence. This includes increasing the capacity of state and local communities to increase their individual and system capacity to engage in prevention activities. DELTA and EMPOWER programs included in this case study used a 10-step planning process called Getting To Outcomes (GTO). For both projects, the prevention planning process was guided by the principles of empowerment evaluation (for an in-depth description of the DELTA and EMPOWER programs, GTO, and empowerment evaluation principles, see Cox, Ortega, Cook-Craig, & Conway, 2010/this issue).

Defining Community Types

The DELTA and EMPOWER states profiled in this case study represent states whose communities are primarily rural, frontier, and geographically isolated. Multiple definitions exist for each of these community types; the definition and distinctions used to define the case study communities are provided below.

Defining rural communities

Although multiple definitions are used to define a rural community, the Census uses a population-based perspective, defining a city, town, or village with a population of 2,500 or fewer as rural (Reynnells, 2008; U.S. Census Bureau, 1994). The current study uses the Census definition. The total population of the EMPOWER state highlighted in this case study, Kentucky, is just more than 4 million people (U.S. Census Bureau, 2000). Kentucky is a state with a high concentration of people living in rural communities (53.9%) (U.S. Census Bureau, 2009). This state is also plagued by persistent poverty, well above the national poverty rate (U.S. Census Bureau, 2000). Communities with high poverty rates are concentrated in the eastern part of the state (see U.S. Census Bureau Small Area Income and Poverty Estimates Program, 2009) where rural communities face greater geographic isolation due the Appalachian mountain chain.

Defining frontier communities

A frontier community is a type of rural community characterized by very low population density. According to the National Center for Frontier Communities (2000), a community is designated as frontier if it has a population density of 20 persons per square mile located more than 60 miles and/or 60 minutes from the nearest market center. Montana, the DELTA state included in this case study, has a significant number of communities that meet the low population density criteria to be designated as frontier. It has a population density of 6.2 people per square mile. The largest city has a population of approximately 90,000 people (U.S. Census Bureau, 2000). Like Kentucky, Montana's poverty rate is also higher than the national average (U.S. Census Bureau, 2000). The state is not in any of the top 100 media markets (Digital Syndicate Network, 2009) and lacks any significant corporate or national foundation's presence. All of these factors necessitate developing more innovative, cost-effective means for building capacity and communication resources in the state.

Defining geographically isolated communities

Although definitions of rural and frontier communities are often based on measurement of population density in a region, many fields have also recognized that communities can face barriers to accessing services due to factors related to geographic or climate conditions and are referred to as geographical isolated (see Leipert & Reutter, 1998, 2005). This designation refers to a type of rural community that not only has a low population density but is also constrained or isolated by specific geographical or climatological features (mountains, rivers, oceans, distance, harsh weather conditions). Kentucky and Montana contain communities that are geographically isolated. For example, one county in Montana is split by a mountain range. Travel in the county for intervention response or for prevention planning meetings is hindered, when roads are impassable, such as in poor weather conditions in the winter. Several communities across Kentucky are separated by mountains, hills, hollers, and lakes. In the eastern region of the state, winter or emergency weather conditions can make mountain roads impassable for weeks or longer.

Community Size and Risk of Violence Perpetration

Individual, relationship, community, and societal level risk factors for IPV and perpetration of SV may be experienced differently by rural, frontier, and geographically isolated communities. For instance, three community-level factors associated with increased risk of IPV and SV, poverty, lack of employment opportunities, and lack of institutional support (Centers for Disease Control and Prevention, 2008, 2009), are found in high proportions in many rural communities. In a recent examination of poverty in rural communities, Albrecht, Albrecht, and Albrecht (2000) found that "poverty is more extensive and more severe in non-metropolitan areas" (p. 87). Lichter and Johnson (2007) suggested that poverty for persons living in rural areas who are minorities is exceptionally high. The extreme poverty in rural areas has been exacerbated by "extensive industrial and economic transformation . . . including an increase in the service-sector employment" (Albrecht et al., 2000, p. 87). Poverty is tied to children's experience with violence (Carlson, 2006; Gelles, 1992). Carlson (2006) found a significant relationship between poverty and youth exposure to violence in rural communities.

Rural communities also struggle with providing adequate institutional support services needed to meet the needs of their populations. Many funding mechanisms associated with community services use population-based funding structures that ensure that rural communities receive fewer resources than areas with higher population counts regardless of the magnitude of the problems they are facing. In addition, services in rural areas are harder to access. For instance, rural women experiencing domestic violence also face more barriers accessing social services and medical help (Hilbert & Krishnan, 2000; Ulbrich & Stockdale, 2002). The fact that rural communities can experience heightened risk of some factors associated with IPV and SV makes the need to include these communities as a part of prevention planning processes critically important.

Promoting Inclusion in Rural and Frontier Violence Prevention Planning

One of the guiding principles behind the DELTA and EMPOWER projects is to promote inclusion of key stakeholders in the violence prevention planning process (for an in-depth description of the DELTA and EMPOWER programs, GTO, and Empowerment Evaluation principles see Cox et al., this issue). Inclusion, as defined by Wandersman et al. (2005), is a commitment to involving stakeholders from all levels and all constituencies. Focusing on inclusion ensures that all community members have an equal voice in planning. By working to create a process that has specific strategies designed to include various constituencies, state and local planners can ensure that historically underserved or disempowered groups are brought into the planning process. In addition, when a planning process is built on a framework that fosters inclusion of all community members, other guiding principles such as fostering community ownership and using local community knowledge become possible.

The principle of inclusion is particularly difficult for rural, frontier, and geographically isolated communities; members face greater challenges in participating in group-planning processes than planning members of urban communities. It is for this reason that this case study examines barriers and solutions to creating inclusion in rural and frontier communities.

Social network theory can provide a useful framework for understanding why inclusiveness in rural communities can be difficult. *Social network theory* refers to the set of assumptions guiding one's understanding of the nature of people's connections with one another (Scott, 2000). Social network theory suggests that, other factors being equal, people are more likely to connect with one another if they are located within geographic proximity to one another, a phenomenon known as propinquity (Kadushin, 2004). The physical isolation of rural communities creates significant barriers to making sure that key stakeholders from all parts of the state are a part of planning processes.

The projects highlighted in this case study placed a high importance on creating a violence prevention planning process that was inclusive but also faced unique challenges based on the rural, frontier, and geographically isolated communities each project contained. The purpose of this case study was to explore the question of what barriers existed for these communities and how those barriers were overcome. A description of the case study methodology and the findings of the current study follow.

METHOD

A case study approach allows for the in-depth examination of a process (Yin, 2003). The current study's goal is to examine how states with primarily rural or frontier communities engaged in an inclusive process to plan for the primary prevention of IPV and SV. This strategy can analyze an individual instance of a phenomenon or a population of cases representing that phenomenon (Stake, 2000). Two instances representing primary prevention planning in rural and frontier states were examined.

Data Collection

Secondary data based on document analysis of publicly-available documents created as part of participation in prevention planning work in both states and synthesis of program experiences drawn from the experiences of empowerment evaluators for each program was used. Examples of documents include project descriptions, information created for state coalition Web sites, prevention plans, and minutes of meetings.

Data Analysis

Documents for each of the two states were analyzed separately using thematic analysis (Boyatzis, 1998) to search for barriers and opportunities associated with increasing inclusivity in the planning process. Results of these individual analyses were integrated together using a cross-case method (Yin, 2003) to compare inclusivity strategies that were common or different across the two states. This resulted in findings associated with barriers to ensuring inclusivity in the prevention planning process, innovative strategies designed to ensure inclusivity used as a part of the two states' planning processes, and opportunities identified that would aid in increasing inclusivity in rural areas. Results common across both states are presented without highlighting a particular program; results specific to one of the cases are presented with specific reference to that state.

Description of the Sample of Cases

Case study state 1: DELTA in a frontier state

Montana is the frontier DELTA state. It focused on preventing initial victimization and perpetration of IPV by building prevention and evaluation capacity at four levels: local, state, organizational, and national. The Montana Coalition Against Domestic and Sexual Violence (MCADSV) began receiving CDC DELTA funding in 2002 and in 2003 started providing resources, funding, training, and technical assistance to local DELTA-funded communities to improve their organizational capacity to prevent IPV. The MCADSV formed a Statewide Steering Committee (SSC) to design a state-level approach to IPV prevention that would reinforce and compliment local prevention strategies. The SSC met face-to-face two to four times per year. The number of face-to-face meetings was limited due to financial constraints associated with the necessary travel required to coalesce a group of stakeholders who represented the diversity of the state. MCADSV also provided training and technical assistance to local teams, called Coordinated Community Response Groups, that worked to implement IPV primary prevention strategies in their local communities.

Case study state 2: EMPOWER in a rural state

Kentucky joined the EMPOWER project in 2005. The project is managed jointly by the Kentucky Department of Health, working in conjunction with the state coalition for SV program (Kentucky Association of Sexual Assault Programs [KASAP]) and the Kentucky Cabinet for Health and Families. The state was asked to join the CDC EMPOWER project but was awarded funding for travel to receive technical assistance only. As such, Kentucky received no funds to develop their prevention plan. Kentucky created a State Prevention Team (SPT), a committee of approximately 30 people representing different stakeholders across the state. The SPT met four times each year, with subcommittees meeting as needed between quarterly SPT meetings. Travel to face-to face meetings was also difficult for this state due to limited funding and geographic proximity constraints.

The synthesis of these two states' experiences suggests that rural states may encounter common barriers and strategies for counteracting these barriers when engaging in prevention planning.

RESULTS

Barriers Associated With Prevention Planning for Rural, Frontier, and Geographically Isolated Communities

Both states experienced similar challenges in creating an inclusive process. Three challenges emerged as particularly important: geography, funding, and access to evidence-based strategies.

Geographic proximity

One of the more obvious barriers to prevention planning for rural states and communities is distance. Social network theory indicates that people will more easily connect if they are geographically close. Because rurality creates natural distance between prevention partners, additional work is created by the need to ensure that the process of planning for the prevention of IPV or SV includes a structure that will allow for participation of all partners, rather than just physically close partners. In rural communities, the simple task of bringing people together can be associated with increased costs in time and money, both to the individual and the organization that is reimbursing travel. In order to ensure meaningful participation of geographically distant partners, specific attention must be paid to the development of strategies to connect people.

In addition, geographical proximity was a consideration when reviewing viable primary prevention strategies and how they can be accessed in rural, frontier, and geographically isolated communities. For example, an assessment of assets in communities in Kentucky showed that assets are allocated regionally and services are provided regionally. This creates a fabric of intervention and prevention services that are physically located in the population center of a region. The impact on individuals and families is that they may have to travel across county lines (and sometimes several counties) to access needed programming (Cook, Morris, & Kelly, 2006). Practitioners from Kentucky were particularly concerned that getting individuals to attend prevention programs would be difficult if they had to travel distances to attend.

Funding challenges

Rural communities also faced increased challenges with regard to securing funding to engage in prevention work. Some funding mechanisms are population-based, such as Rape, Prevention, and Education funds administered by the CDC, which leaves rural, less densely populated communities with less funding than communities with a high population density. Tasks associated with primary prevention planning as in GTO are the same regardless of the level of funding states and their local communities receive. Less funding means less ability to pay for staff, volunteer committee members' travel, and other costs associated with prevention planning. Rural communities, who may have a high level of motivation to participate in planning processes, may be forced to shoulder higher costs associated with travel but with less money. Strategies to include rural partners must therefore address the question of the cost-effectiveness of solutions to increase inclusion.

Access to evidence

Part of the GTO planning process includes searching for evidence-based strategies to prevent the perpetration of violence. However, rural, frontier, and geographically isolated communities may not have adequate access to research databases where such literature is housed. The planning partners in these two states experienced increased burdens associated with connecting to university and public libraries where access to such databases exists. Although many journals provide online access to articles, it is often associated with membership or high fees for one-time article access, making access by individual rural community partners or rural organization to evidence-based literature a costly proposition.

Two other factors associated with access to evidence are important to note. First, one criticism of the reliance of evidence-based strategies in the strategy selection process is that for many societal problems, there is a lack of evidence to suggest which strategies are most effective (Johnson & Austin, 2006; Reid, Kenaley, & Colvin, 2004; Rosen, Proctor, & Staudt, 1999). This is true of the prevention of perpetration of IPV and SV (Casey & Linshorst, 2009). States participating in the EMPOWER and DELTA programs found it necessary to examine strategies that were evidence informed or were promising (based on program evaluation findings) due to the lack of available evidence-based strategies.

A second and related challenge for rural communities in prevention planning processes is that, even for strategies that have research evidence suggesting effectiveness, they are almost always evaluated with groups of people from nonrural populations. In a recent review of primary prevention approaches to decrease sexual assault perpetration, Casey and Linshorst (2009) found only two programs that showed promising evidence of affecting rates of perpetration (Foshee et al., 2004; Foubert, Newberry, & Tatum, 2007). Neither addressed the effectiveness on rural populations. So rural partners face an additional burden of assessing whether evidence-based strategies can be adapted to the local culture of their communities and maintain fidelity to the program due to the lack evaluation research on the implementation of these programs to rural or frontier populations.

Strategies Used to Promote Inclusion

Given these challenges, the two states identified and employed four strategies to ensure that partners from rural, frontier, and geographically isolated communities could meaningfully participate in prevention planning activities.

Using rurality as a lens when creating a planning process

By acknowledging that geography affects the planning process, states were able to infuse knowledge about the unique challenges that potential community partners face into designing the membership, protocols that would facilitate the prevention planning process for the state and its local communities. One strategy used to design an inclusive planning team was conducting an assessment on how rural partners have participated in past state and local planning efforts. This allowed for recruitment of a planning team that included those needed at the table rather than just those usually at the table. A broader list of potential planning partners emerged. For example, schools and faith communities often are the main (and sometimes only) social centers in rural communities. Representatives from these groups at the prevention planning table are valuable; they can report on the concerns, the pulse of rural residents. Geographical representation can then be used as a variable that is accounted for in developing a final list of planning partners.

Once planning team partners were selected, paying attention to local resources that planning team members from rural communities brought helped identify their roles on the planning team. For instance, team members with low access to databases may not have the tools they need to assist with searching for potential evidence-based strategies. They did have access to local data and knowledge of local community resources and connections and relationships. They were crucial to working on adapting strategies to address the local culture of the communities.

In addition to using a rurality lens to create a planning team, it was also used to create the structure for moving the planning process forward. Understanding challenges rural planning partners faced helped guide decisions about when, where, how often, and why the team met face-to-face. Explicit discussions of what tasks needed to be completed in the room with other partners in light of these challenges were useful in increasing the likelihood of member participation and in promoting a culture of inclusion with the team. In addition, the use of a rurality lens affected how funds available for planning processes are used. By acknowledging the increased expenses that rural partners incur to participate, the planning team set aside funds to pay for costs associated with participation to ease the burden that rural partners experience in getting to meetings.

USING RURALITY AS A DIMENSION IN THE PLANNING PROCESS

In addition to infusing knowledge about rurality into the design of the planning process, rurality was used as a dimension in the completion of planning tasks. This was particularly useful in completing the state profile, creating goal and outcome statements, and in reviewing evidence prevention strategies for the needs assessment. Part of completing the prevention plan included creating state and local community profiles. Paying attention to the ways that rural areas define *community* allowed the planning team to create profiles that were meaningful to the constituencies involved. The process of crafting goals and outcome statements provided another opportunity to address rural needs. Kentucky's team explicitly included developing access to prevention programming to rural communities as a goal in the plan.

Available research evidence had to be translated for the practitioner to be meaningfully applied to practice. A major issue identified in the literature is the lack of effective strategies that guide the implementation of evidence in practice (Fixsen, Naoom, Blase, Friedman, & Wallace, 2005; Mullen, Bledsoe, & Bellamy, 2008). With respect to rural communities, little or no literature addresses how evidence-based and evidence-informed strategies apply to the local cultures of rural communities. This heightens the importance of providing training and technical assistance to communities on strategy adaption, because most rural communities will be adapting selected strategies to local cultural conditions.

USING WEB TECHNOLOGY AND INFORMATION TECHNOLOGY TO PROMOTE INCLUSION

In the DELTA and EMPOWER projects, the use of technology was a very effective strategy to increase participation and inclusion of rural team members. It was important to identify ways that rural or isolated partners in each state could be involved, maximizing their expertise in a time-efficient and cost-effective manner. When possible face-to-face meetings were replaced with Web-based conference calls to allow for increased participation. When face-to-face meetings occurred and rural partners were unable to attend, they actively communicated via a Web-based conferencing system such as Skype or by conference call. One challenge of working with planning groups via conference calls is that not all participants find this an effective (or even an accessible) learning venue. Some participants were better visual learners.

In Montana, planners established a Website where call participants could view PowerPoint presentations, agendas, and other visual aids during the calls. This technology tended to increase interest and sustain engagement.

Some participants spoke readily and often, but it was difficult to gauge the level of understanding of silent partners. Using another Website feature, participants could choose to submit written comments or questions during the call. The Website also helped fill the database gap by including documents and links of otherwise locally, hard-to-access information.

At each stage of the planning process, steering committee members formed workgroups/teams to complete specific tasks or sections; for example, Montana created a Need Statements Team, Goals Teams for specific goals or groups of goals,; and a Format and Dissemination of the Public Plan Team. The team leader convened the group and communicated recommendations to the full team, using e-mail and conference calls. Web and information technology (IT) resources also were used to build the capacity of steering committee members and planning groups in the DELTA communities in Montana. The focus was on providing replicable trainings and tools to be used by the local communities to increase their capacity to engage in primary prevention planning and strategies. Members received articles, resource lists, Website links, summary sheets, bibliographies, PowerPoint presentations, games, and discussion/training aids via a Resources CD and via e-mail. The coalition's lending library was a ready source at no cost. Using their Web-based library catalogue, members could conduct a search for materials and submit a loan request. A listserv to exchange information and as a means of posting synopses of pertinent primary prevention and evaluation literature was created. Employing these strategies to make resources available, it broadened the opportunities to access resources often unavailable in small communities.

In Kentucky the use of the Web and e-mail was important for the state planning team to engage in document review and writing. This allowed members to respond to and engage in document creation and editing even if they were unable to attend face-to-face meetings. In addition, it maximized inclusion of partners who may have been unwilling or unable to voice their concerns or share their expertise in large group face-to-face meeting but felt more comfortable responding to documents online.

ALTERNATIVE METHODS FOR INPUT BY LOCAL PARTNERS IN THE PLANNING PROCESS

One primary method for involvement of rural community members in the process was to invite them to join as members of the planning committee, as in Montana. In Kentucky a committee of local community partners formed as a subcommittee of the state coalition for sexual assault programs to work in partnership with the state prevention team around the issue of strategy selection.

Montana demonstrated another way to ensure inclusion of partners from rural communities, inviting them to provide regular reports and discussions at face-to-face steering committee meetings. This became a way to ensure their voice in the process, but accommodated the challenges they faced to attend more regular meetings.

Opportunities Associated With Prevention Planning for Rural Communities

The process of prevention planning offered Montana the opportunity to express their independent and self-sufficient identity. Most representatives of the state planning committee in Montana lived in a rural setting and were aware of the barriers and opportunities in such communities. Living in a low population state, they were more likely to personally know or know someone who knows important parties to include at the table. In analyzing this case it became clear that the empowerment evaluation (EE) process had a special appeal for citizens of frontier and predominantly rural states who tend to think of themselves as independent and self-sufficient, because, as the theorists of EE stated, the purpose is to "use evaluation concepts, techniques, and findings to foster improvement and self-determination" (Fetterman, 1996, p. 4).

This process also created a new mandate within both states to think about ways of bringing statewide stakeholders together. The challenge of inclusion was not one of finding committed stakeholders but of solving logistical constraints. The decision by each state to participate in DELTA and EMPOWER necessitated that the states revisit who was involved in violence prevention planning in the state and what difficulties are associated with participation in the task. This process afforded the states the opportunity to engage these partners in problem solving about how to get together to do this work and to try new strategies for including needed partners.

DISCUSSION

As described in this case study, the goal of encouraging an inclusive process that encouraged maximum participation by local and state stakeholders in violence prevention planning was a difficult but rewarding one. The decision by the CDC to use EE as a guiding philosophical framework for the DELTA and EMPOWER projects was an important foundation for establishing inclusion as guiding principle from which states should do their prevention work. This set the tone for the DELTA and EMPOWER states in this case study to focus on addressing the needs of partners who traditionally experience barriers in participating in state and community planning processes. For organizations that provide services to families, this is an important focus. To the extent that planning teams can decrease the significant barriers that providers and prevention partners face in participating in prevention planning, the likelihood that rural partners will participate is increased.

The use of technology to connect geographically distant or isolated partners is becoming a popular strategy to promote inclusion. One European study suggests that, though participants in technologically based learning and training programs in geographically isolated communities do not often get the opportunity to participate in these programs, the majority are open, very interested, or extremely interested in future participation (Tiropanis, Tsekeridou, Serif, Stergioulas, & Ghinea, 2007). Kentucky and Montana's experience suggests that technology was a key factor in participation for isolated partners.

The recognition that the assumptions of social network theory tell us that the natural inclination is to connect with partners that are geographically close to us was also an important consideration in increasing inclusiveness of rural partners. This recognition created a planning process that actively sought to develop mechanisms and structures that resisted this inclination and explicitly sought to decrease barriers that naturally impede the participation of rural partners. Acknowledging the assumptions behind social network theory and the role that geographical proximity plays in developing collaborative teams, those building prevention planning teams can recognize that important partners may not have been included in past prevention strategy-building processes.

Funding partners could support this process by looking for opportunities to include funding to engage rural partners using technological resources. The use of technology made a positive difference in these two projects; however, this strategy can only be used when agencies and planning teams have the funding to execute it. By incorporating money for access to technology in their funding mechanisms, funding partners can make a tangible contribution to prevention planning teams in their efforts to include rural partners.

Implications for Family Social Work

Family social workers in rural communities face challenges in connecting with one another that may contribute to feelings of professional isolation and a lack of confidence that systems change is possible. What may be required is the recognition that not only are rural families and individuals who experience violence isolated from help (Hilbert & Krishnan, 2000; Ulbrich & Stockdale, 2002); however, professionals can be isolated as well. This case study suggests greater use of technology can provide a meaningful avenue for family social workers to work together to promote capacity building and systems change related to prevention.

In addition, it is important for agencies that work with victims and perpetrators of violence provide structural support for family social workers to plan together. This support must come in the form of funding, time, and technological infrastructure necessary to meet face-to-face and via other mechanisms.

Directions for Future Research

Although this case study suggests that there are strategies that can promote inclusion of partners in rural communities for violence prevention programming, much more research is needed to expand the knowledge base about how this can optimally be achieved. By intentionally and creatively looking for ways to address the unique needs of organizations and prevention partners from rural communities, the two DELTA and EMPOWER states were able to increase the likelihood that voices from across each state were included in the prevention planning process. However, the impact of the use of these strategies and techniques needs to be researched further. As the DELTA and EMPOWER projects move forward to complete the final steps of the GTO process, replicating evaluations of the use of technological resources to connect rural partners (for an example, see Tiropanis et al., 2007) would be useful in gaining quantitative data on how these resources impact members participation in the project. In addition, quantitative research is needed to assess the impact that such actions have on prevention program outcomes.

REFERENCES

Albrecht, D. E., Albrecht, C. M., & Albrecht, S. L. (2000). Poverty in non-metropolitan America: Impacts of industrial, employment, and family structure variables. *Rural Sociology, 65*, 87–103.

Boyatzis, R. E. (1998). *Transforming qualitative information: Thematic analysis and code development.* Thousand Oaks, CA: Sage.

Carlson, K. T. (2006). Poverty and youth violence exposure: Experiences in rural communities. *Children & Schools, 28*, 87–96.

Casey, E. A., & Linshorst, T. P. (2009). Toward a multi-level, ecological approach to the primary prevention of sexual assault: Prevention in peer and community contexts. *Trauma, Violence, and Abuse, 10*, 91–114.

Centers for Disease Control and Prevention. (2008, October 21). *Intimate partner violence: Risk and protective factors.* Retrieved from http://www.cdc.gov/ViolencePrevention/intimatepartnerviolence/riskprotectivefactors.html

Centers for Disease Control and Prevention. (2009, January 27). *Sexual violence: Risk and protective factors.* Retrieved from http://www.cdc.gov/ViolencePrevention/sexualviolence/riskprotectivefactors.html

Cook, P. G., Morris, F., & Kelly, N. (2006). *Kentucky statewide violence prevention strategic plan.* Frankfort, KY: Cabinet for Health and Families.

Cox, P., Ortega, S., Cook-Craig, P. G., & Conway, P. (2010). Strengthening systems for the primary prevention of sexual violence and intimate partner violence: CDC's DELTA and EMPOWER programs. *Journal of Family Social Work, 13*(4), 287–296.

Digital Syndicate Network. (2009). *Top 100 media markets.* Retrieved from http://www.digitalsyndicate.tv/markets.html

Fetterman, D. M. (1996). Empowerment evaluation. In D. M. Fetterman, S. J. Kaftarian, & A. Wandersman (Eds.), *Empowerment evaluation: Knowledge and tools for self-assessment & accountability* (pp. 3–46). Thousand Oaks, CA: Sage.

Fixsen, D. L., Naoom, S. F., Blase, K. A., Friedman, R. M., & Wallace, F. (2005). *Implementation research: A synthesis of the literature*. Tampa, FL: The National Implementation Research Network.

Foshee, V. A., Bauman, K. E., Ennett, S. T., Fletcher-Linder, G., Benefield, T., & Suchindran, C. (2004). Assessing the long-term effects of the Safe Dates Program and a booster in preventing and reducing adolescent dating violence victimization and perpetration. *American Journal of Public Health, 94*, 619–624.

Foubert, J. D., Newberry, J. T., & Tatum, J. L. (2007). Behavior differences seven months later: Effects of a rape prevention program on first-year men who join fraternities. *NASPA Journal, 44*, 728–749.

Gelles, R. J. (1992). Poverty and violence toward children. *American Behavioral Scientist, 35*, 258–274.

Hilbert, J. C., & Krishnan, S. P. (2000). Addressing barriers to community care of battered women in rural environments: Creating a policy of social inclusion. *Journal of Health & Social Policy, 12*, 41–52.

Johnson, M., & Austin, M. J. (2006). Evidence-based practice on the social services: Implications for organizational change. *Administration in Social Work, 30*, 75–104.

Kadushin, C. (2004). Some basic network concepts and propositions. In *Introduction to social network theory*. Retrieved from http://stat.gamma.rug.nl/snijders/Kadushin_Concepts.pdf

Leipurt, B. D., & Reuttner, L. (1998). Women's health and community health nursing practice in geographically isolated settings: A Canadian perspective. *Health Care for Women International, 19*, 575–588.

Leipurt, B. D., & Reuttner, L. (2005). Developing resilience: How women maintain their health in northern geographically isolated settings. *Qualitative Health Research, 15*, 49–65.

Lichter, D. T., & Johnson, K. M. (2007). The changing spatial concentration of America's rural poor population. *Rural Sociology, 72*, 331–358.

Mullen, E. J., Bledsoe, S. E., & Bellamy, J. L. (2008). Implementing evidence-based social work practice. *Research on Social Work Practice, 18*, 325–338.

National Center for Frontier Communities. (2000). *2000 update: Frontier counties in the United States*. Retrieved from http://www.frontierus.org/2000update.htm

Reid, W. J., Kenaley, B. D., & Colvin, J. (2004). Do some interventions work better than others? A review of comparative social work experiments? *Social Work Research, 28*(2), 71–82.

Reynnells, L. (2008). *What is rural?* USDA National Agricultural Library Rural Information Center. Retrieved from http://www.nal.usda.gov/ric/ricpubs/what_is_rural.shtml

Rosen, A., Proctor, E. K., & Staudt, M. M. (1999). Social work research and the quest for effective practice. *Social Work Research, 23*, 4–14.

Scott, J. (2000). *Social network analysis: A handbook*. Thousand Oaks, CA: Sage.

Stake, R. E. (2000). Case studies. In N. K. Denzin & Y. S. Lincoln (Eds.), *Handbook of qualitative research* (2nd ed., pp. 435–454). Thousand Oaks, CA: Sage.

Tiropanis, T., Tsekeridou, S., Serif, T., Stergioulas, L., & Ghinea, G. (2007). *Empowering geographically isolated communities with instant access to learning and training through satellite*. Paper presented at the EDEN 2007 Annual Conference, Naples, Italy. Retrieved from http://eprints.soton.ac.uk/50020/

Ulbrich, P. M., & Stockdale, J. (2002). Making family planning clinics an empowerment zone for rural battered women. *Women & Health*, *35*(2/3), 83–100.

U.S. Census Bureau. (1994). The urban and rural classifications. In U.S. Department of Commerce Economics and Statistics Administration (Ed.), *Geographic areas reference manual* (pp. 12.1–12.24). Retrieved from http://www.census.gov/geo/www/GARM/Ch12GARM.pdf

U.S. Census Bureau. (2000). *American factfinder*. U.S. Census Bureau. Retrieved from http://factfinder.census.gov/servletDatabaseMainPageServlet?_program=DEC&_SubmenuID=&_lang=en&_ts=

U.S. Census Bureau Small Area Income and Poverty Estimates (SAIPE) Program. (2009). *Percent in poverty, 2008*. U.S. Census Bureau. Retrieved from http://www.census.gov/did/www/saipe/data/statecounty/maps/iy2008/Tot_Pct_Poor2008.pdf

Wandersman, A., Snell-Johns, J., Lentz, B., Fetterman, D. M., Keener, D. C., Livet, M., et al. (2005). The principles of empowerment evaluation. In D. M. Fetterman & A. Wandersman (Eds.), *Empowerment evaluation principles in practice* (pp. 27–41). New York: Guilford Press.

Yin, L. (2003). *Case study research: Design and methods* (3rd ed.). Thousand Oaks, CA: Sage.

Using Empowerment Evaluation to Facilitate the Development of Intimate Partner and Sexual Violence Prevention Programs

PAT CONWAY
School of Medicine and Health Sciences, University of North Dakota, Grand Forks, North Dakota

JANET CRESSWELL
Women's Action and Resource Center, Beulah, North Dakota

DIANE HARMON
Domestic Violence Crisis Center, Minot, North Dakota

CHARLES POSPISHIL
School of Medicine and Health Sciences, University of North Dakota, Grand Forks, North Dakota

KATHY SMITH
Rape and Abuse Crisis Center, Fargo, North Dakota

JENNIFER WAGES
School of Medicine and Health Sciences, University of North Dakota, Grand Forks, North Dakota

LISA WEISZ
Women's Action and Resource Center, Beulah, North Dakota

This article addresses the question, "What factors contributed to successful completion of a needs and resource assessment in local communities, using the empowerment evaluation approach?" Case studies of three successful projects allow the exploration of organizational, community, state, and national factors that contributed to a strong needs and resource assessment, including original data collection, to guide the development of a plan to prevent intimate partner and sexual violence. The overall project was guided by empowerment evaluation principles. Each local community used additional conceptual frameworks, including grounded theory, Kolberg's theory of moral development, gender-role attitudes as operationalized by the rape myth acceptance and Olweis' systemic approach to bullying. Local programs focused on specific populations and collected original data through a variety of methods. For instance, one local agency utilized already existing surveys to assess bullying within their public school setting. Another community assessed the attitudes of male sex offenders and other male community members regarding gender-role attitudes, violence, and risk and protective factors for perpetration. A third community administered a random phone survey, examining attitudes toward rape, other violence against women, and gender roles. Each community integrated the results of their original data collection into their needs and resource assessment. Preliminary information regarding the communities' experience with the completion of needs and resource assessments, using the empowerment evaluation framework, indicate that successful projects used specific theories or frameworks to guide data collection. Positive collaboration with evaluators and community prevention coalitions characterized each community's experience.

Prevention programs designed to reduce the incidence of intimate partner violence (IPV) and sexual violence (SV) are relatively new in the United States. In 2000, the Centers for Disease Control and Prevention's (CDC) National Center for Injury Prevention and Control embarked on an effort to develop primary prevention priorities for IPV, stating that the focus previously had been on secondary and tertiary prevention (National Center for Injury Prevention and Control, 2002). Given the high rates of violence against women, an estimated 40% to 60% of women experience IPV at some point in their lifetime (Coulter, 2004), one in six women experience rape (Tjaden & Thoennes, 1998), primary prevention is essential. The current study presents three rural, upper midwestern communities' stories of their implementation of one model for prevention of IPV and SV, Getting To Outcomes and empowerment evaluation. Developed and funded by the CDC, North Dakota created its statewide project, the North Dakota Intimate Partner and Sexual Violence Prevention Project. Eleven local communities were selected to participate, five with a combined IPV and SV prevention project, five with SV prevention programming only, and one with IPV prevention programming only. This ambitious undertaking required that local communities who had primarily focused on interventions with victims of IPV and SV think and work in new ways. This article presents the story of three local programs whose communities successfully implemented the first step of their prevention program, completion of a needs and resource (N&R) assessment, to identify factors that contributed to their success and ways in which challenges were addressed.

The Bioecological Approach

The North Dakota Intimate Partner and Sexual Violence Prevention Project operated under the tenets of the bioecological approach, addressing multiple systems levels, individual, family, community, and broader society (Bronfenbrenner & Ceci, 1994). This model proposes that individual behavior results from biological forces, including genetic predispositions and environmental influences. To understand human behavior and prevent undesirable outcomes, one must address varied system levels. For instance, reducing perpetration would mean changing the behavior of an individual who is violent, and the factors that predispose that individual to violence, such as early childhood experiences and gender-role norms (Bohner, Siebler, & Schmelcher, 2006).

Empowerment Evaluation

Community-based participatory action research, which has a central premise that data collection begins at the local level and involves persons who are the subject of the research (Bordeaux et al., 2007), provides the basis for empowerment evaluation, the model undergirding the North Dakota Intimate Partner and Sexual Violence Prevention Project at the state and local levels (Fetterman & Wandersman, 2005). Empowerment evaluation has been used in a number of other prevention projects, notably prevention of substance abuse (Fetterman, Kaftarian, & Wandersman, 1995). Its 10 principles are improvement, community ownership, inclusion, democratic participation, social justice, community knowledge, evidenced-based strategies, capacity building, organizational learning, and accountability (Fetterman et al., 1995; see Cox, Ortega, Cook-Craig, & Conway, 2010/this issue for description of empowerment evaluation). The intended outcome of empowerment evaluation processes is a change in power (Miller & Campbell, 2006). Research regarding the efficacy of empowerment evaluation is mixed (Chinman, Imm, & Wandersman, 2004; Fetterman & Wandersman, 2005). Fidelity to the principles is difficult to maintain for a variety of reasons; agency readiness is particularly critical to an agency's ability to follow empowerment evaluation (Fetterman & Wandersman, 2005; Miller & Campbell, 2006).

Getting To Outcomes (GTO), paired with empowerment evaluation, provided the structure guiding the prevention work in the project to prevent IPV and SV in local communities across North Dakota (see Cox, Ortega, Cook-Craig, & Conway, 2010/this issue for a description of GTO). The first step in the GTO process is conducting a comprehensive N&R assessment, followed by development of goals, outcomes, and activities. A community coalition guides the process, bringing widespread involvement, knowledge, and expertise. The resulting information from program evaluation is intended to be used for program development and sustainability. This complex project, with national, state, and local components, has potential for positive change in families across the state and in other communities where similar prevention work is emerging. Its promise and challenges are described here through the experiences of three communities.

METHOD

This multiple case study (Yin, 2003) describes the experiences of three communities, to identify factors that contributed to their successful implementation of GTO Step 1, conducting a N&R assessment, based on empowerment evaluation principles, and challenges they experienced.

Sample

The three communities, ranging in size from 8,600 in the smallest county to a midsized community of 37,000 to the largest community in the state at 100,000, were selected based on their success in completing their local N&R assessment. The communities focused on specific populations and collected original data through a variety of quantitative and qualitative methods. For instance, one local agency utilized already existing surveys to assess bullying within their public school setting. Another community assessed the attitudes of male community members regarding gender-role attitudes, violence, and factors that are risk and protective factors for perpetration. A third administered a random phone survey, examining attitudes toward rape, other violence against women, and gender roles. Each community integrated the results of their original data collection into their N&R assessment and used the information to guide the development of their prevention program.

Characteristics of the sample

The three communities have very different local IPV and SV organizations. In addition to differences in staff size, two of the three programs focused on prevention of SV, one on prevention of SV and IPV. All three participated in a statewide program that provided technical assistance regarding empowerment evaluation, GTO, and primary prevention of IPV and SV.

Case 1: Mercer County Women's Action Resource Center (WARC) of Beulah, in western North Dakota, provides direct services to victims of IPV and SV. It serves a rural county of approximately 8,600 people; the county is unique in that it has a significantly higher per capita income due to the presence of several electric generating power plants whose skilled labor force raises the average compensation level.

Case 2: The Domestic Violence Crisis Center (DVCC) provides services to victims of IPV in Ward County, north central North Dakota, the regional trade center. Ward County is a predominantly urban county of 58,795 people. Minot, where the DVCC is located, is its largest community. The Minot area has a 4-year state university and a U.S. Air Force Base.

Case 3: The Rape and Abuse Crisis Center (RACC) is a nonprofit agency that provides crisis intervention, advocacy, and counseling services for persons affected by IPV and SV. The RACC also provides education and prevention programs to end violence in society. The RACC serves Cass County in southeastern North Dakota, a predominantly urban county. Cass County has a population of 123,138 people; 86.6% of the population of Cass County resides in the cities of Fargo and West Fargo. The Fargo Metro area is a regional trade center in the upper Midwest. It contains a large public university as well as several smaller colleges and trade schools. Cass County is also noted for having a significant immigrant and refugee population.

Statewide intimate partner and sexual violence program

North Dakota, with 640,000 residents, is projected to decrease in population between 2000 and 2010; it has 9.3 persons per square mile, compared with the national rate of 79.6 per square mile (U.S. Census Bureau, 2009). The fastest growing age group is persons older than age 65 years. American Indian and Alaska Native persons constitute 5.4% of the population, up from 3.08% in 1980. They are, on average, younger than the total population (22.6 years American Indian; 37.4 years White) (University of North Dakota, 2004). The North Dakota Intimate Partner and Sexual Violence Prevention Program, managed by the North Dakota IPV and SV program and the state's department of health, combined funding from Rape Prevention Education and the CDC's Domestic Violence Prevention Enhancements and Leadership Through Alliances (DELTA), and Enhancing and Making Programs Work to End Rape (EMPOWER) programs to support a state coalition. It also funded local programs that were to use the empowerment evaluation and GTO framework for developing local prevention programming. The combined project, begun in 2006, was characterized by intensive technical assistance from federal and state staff, including evaluation specialists.

Data Collection and Analysis

Data used to create the case studies were obtained from several sources: (1) stories written by each of the three communities; (2) written documents created as part of the implementation of the project at the federal, state, and local levels; (3) observation and personal experience; and 4) a focus group with staff from the three programs. The authors, involved with the project from different perspectives, brought their own wisdom and biases to the project. Staff from the three projects, two empowerment evaluators, and a local coalition member combined their knowledge and experience to create the case studies. Because all authors had a personal investment in the prevention of IPV and SV program, this article reflects those different views. Borrowing from Gilgun, Daly, and Handel (1992), we balanced "role demands" of authorship with "self-demands" of our personal commitment to the project. This issue of balancing demands enriched the discussions between authors.

The team of authors discussed the project first. Then, the three program staff wrote a description of their individual project, based on Yin's (2003) case study method and Steckler and Linnan's (2002) process evaluation models (see Table 1). This information was used in two ways, to (1) summarize the project's experiences and (2) identify factors that contributed to the three community's successes. The three program staff then participated in a focus group, where a conversation ensued about commonalities and differences across the projects. Three authors, the empowerment evaluators, and coalition members then reviewed the notes from the focus group and the

TABLE 1 Guide for Writing Case Study and Focus Group Conversation

Introduction	1. What is the purpose of project in your local community? 2. How does this project relate to your organization's mission?
Description of community and local coalition	1. Describe your community. Population, rural/urban? Colleges? Any significant demographic factors such as age, race, income, etc. 2. Describe your local coalition. How were members selected? What worked, didn't work? Who became leaders? Did the group change? 3. How did your community react to your project? Was your community ready for change to prevention? What/who were your supports? What were the barriers?
Description of process for conducting N&R assessment and method for data collection	1. What were your feelings when you were told you would be completing a N&R assessment? 2. How was your local coalition involved in your N&R assessment? 3. What was the empowerment evaluator's involvement in your N&R assessment? 4. How did you come up with your data collection plan? 5. Who participated in the data collection? 6. What was successful, not successful?
Results of local program	1. What did the data tell you? 2. What occurred as a result of the data collection?

Note: N&R = needs and resource.

stories to (1) summarize each of the case studies, (2) identify factors contributing to success, and (3) describe to complete the cross case analysis (Yin, 2003).

RESULTS

The three communities, participants in the North Dakota Intimate Partner and Sexual Violence Prevention Project, successfully completed Step 1 of GTO, creating a community N&R assessment regarding prevention of IPV and SV prevention. To accomplish this, they created a community coalition, participated in training and technical assistance, and collected original data. What led to each organization's capacity to successfully complete their N&R assessment, which they then used to develop a SV prevention plan? To document their successes, each community's "story" is presented, using the case study method (Yin, 2003; see Table 1). Factors that contributed to their success and concomitant challenges, identified through the case studies and the focus group, are highlighted.

Case 1

Introduction

When the WARC began their prevention project, they perceived a good fit between it and their agency goal, providing information and resources to empower individuals to choose a life free of violence. They set a prevention goal to increase community knowledge of the nature and extent of SV in their community, as well as risk and protective factors and resources available to combat it. The three staff were committed to this project but felt somewhat out of their element, because they worked in an agency providing direct services to clients, often under an emergency basis. Developing a N&R assessment and focusing on prevention required adaptation.

Description of local coalition

The agency made use of already existing relationships to develop their Sexual Violence Prevention Task Force. Invitations were sent to representatives from Boys & Girl Scouts, the Health Department, and the U.S. Department of Agriculture's local Cooperative Extension Service, as well as middle and high school counselors and the local newspaper. Knowledgeable about their community, the coalition was able to work well together. Despite each member's interest, some were not able to attend coalition meetings regularly. This difficulty was overcome through e-mail communication. After an initial assessment, the coalition reached consensus: their focus would be bullying in the local middle school. Several children had reported being bullied and sexually harassed, potential precursors to sexual and family violence (Basile, Espelage, Rivers, McMahon, & Simon, 2009).

Description of process for conducting needs and resource assessment: method

The coalition based their model for prevention of bullying on the Olweis model, which is congruent with empowerment evaluation principles and systems theory, addressing multiple systems levels, individual, family, and school, and changing power (Olweis, 1993). Its principles are creating (1) a "warm" school and home environment, (2) firm limits on unacceptable behavior, (3) consistent sanctions, and (4) adults as authorities (p. 114). The coalition developed surveys for students, parents, and school staff, addressing the prevalence of and attitudes toward bullying.

Examples of results

The survey of students, staff, and parents found that teasing occurred most days for 28% of the children responding; 20% were physically hurt most days (see Figure 1). The surveys revealed that bullying was a pervasive problem, with most students (66.5%) reporting some sort of bullying. Bullying was not limited to one subset of the population but was pervasive in the community. The current study provided the basis for developing SV prevention plan encompassing a comprehensive antibullying curriculum in the middle school.

Case 2

Introduction

The DVCC, which offers a full range of services to victims of IPV and sexual assault, employed a sexual assault advocate to provide services to survivors,

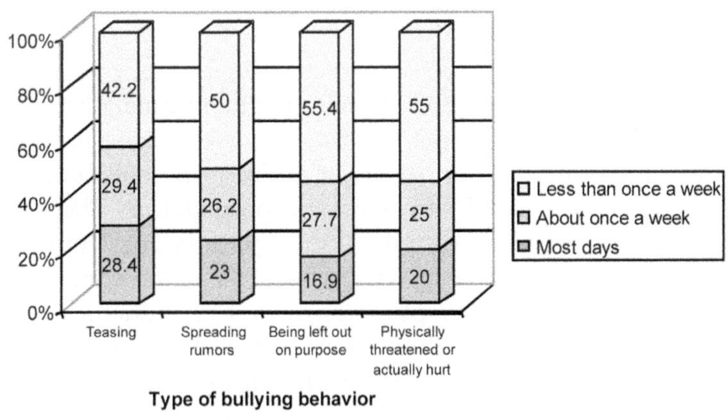

FIGURE 1 Rates of bullying.

including emergency services, advocacy, and support groups. Over the past 3 years, the agency has been moving into prevention programming. Conducting a N&R assessment was a helpful initial step. Although the advocate realized her region had a problem with SV, she was initially overwhelmed by the prospect of conducting the N&R assessment and unsure about what to expect. Because the purpose of the new project was to prevent SV in the community by understanding the nature and extent of the problem and to learn what can be done as a community to confront the issue, the advocate wanted to understand the risk and protective factors: why some men commit sexual offenses and others do not. Grounded theory, an inductive approach beginning with qualitative data collection, identification of themes and hypotheses, and testing those hypotheses, guided the advocate (Gilgun et al., 1992; Glaser & Strauss, 1967). This iterative process continued until she and her local prevention coalition were convinced that no new information was being obtained, the new information led to the discovery of the unexpected, and it facilitated moving in a new direction.

Description of local coalition

The first step in conducting the N&R assessment was to assemble a coalition to conduct the N&R assessment. The Minot Mayor's Safe Community's Group was approached for support, and some members from this group became coalition members. Other members of the coalition included professionals working in SV, college students, and community members who were interested in SV prevention. In addition, members of the Sexual Assault Survivor's Group provided critical input. Two men recommended by the empowerment evaluator to conduct a focus group continued on as coalition members. The advocate built on existing relationships and developed new ones as she built the coalition.

Description of process for conducting needs and resource assessment: method

The first step in the N&R assessment was to obtain information from a Sexual Assault Survivor's Group, who put together a questionnaire for members of local outpatient sexual offender treatment groups. The collaboration served the treatment needs of sexual survivor's and perpetrators. The next step in data collection was a qualitative study of local professionals and community leaders to receive their input regarding issues of SV in the community, assessing community readiness. Attempts were made to conduct focus groups in the community. When this was not successful, individual interviews were used to obtain more information. The coalition used information from the individual interviews and the feedback from the sexual survivors' and sexual offenders' groups to develop a preliminary survey of men in the community.

This survey was piloted with a group of day laborers, who provided feedback regarding the survey's construction. After this process, men in the community, including those in the sexual offender treatment program and men in an anger management program, were surveyed. This survey was analyzed to understand issues in the local community regarding SV and related risk factors. In addition to the use of grounded theory to guide the development of the data collection efforts, the coalition used theory to guide the data analysis. For instance, Kohlberg's theory was used to categorize responses to the question (Daeg de Mott, 2009).

Examples of results

Data analysis and dissemination of the resulting information occurred at each step in the interative process of conducting the N&R assessment. One example of successful collection and dissemination of data was the results of the sex offender treatment group survey; members identified their family as the most important factor contributing to their behavior (see Table 2). In a follow-up survey, this group was more likely than other groups to say their home environment growing up was unsafe, $F(4, 144) = 6.69$, $p = .000$.

The coalition used the results of each stage of data collection to guide program planning. For instance, because different groups were functioning at different stages of development, the coalition determined that prevention strategies needed to vary, so they were appropriate to each of the different levels of moral development. The community survey found that men in the sexual perpetration and anger management groups were most similar: they grew up in violent homes and were more likely to have been abused

TABLE 2 Influences During Childhood

Item	*N*
Positive Influences	13
Family	8
Faith	1
Peers	1
Values	1
Mentor	1
Activities	1
Negative influences	8
Family	5
Peers	1
Viewed as "good kid"	1
Substance abuse	1
Unspecified (positive or negative)	8
Family	3
Media	3
Harsh parenting style	1
Faith	1

as children. The coalition determined that, for younger men, prevention efforts needed to be directed at the influence of the media. This group was exposed to and consumed pornography at a higher rate than other groups, and they appeared at risk because of their indiscriminate use of the media. The same group did not see women as being portrayed inappropriately in advertising.

The results of the N&R assessment have been shared through community forums such as Sexual Assault Awareness Month activities. The results also shaped the goals for their local prevention plan, focusing on strengthening family bonds.

Case 3

Introduction

The RACC, in addition to providing direct services to victims of IPV and SV, has a long history of providing SV prevention programs. In 1980, the agency published the Red Flag Green Flag program, a widely used SV prevention program for children. The RACC has established a relationship with schools in their county to provide IPV and SV prevention programs. Because these programs meet the bench marks established for the North Dakota Counseling Curriculum, the school's buy-in was high.

Description of local coalition

The RACC began working with the DELTA Program in 2004. The agency had already established a coordinated community response coalition (CCR) team, composed of representatives from local law enforcement; the State's Attorney's office, and various social service and public health agencies. The coordinator appointed to conduct the N&R assessment experienced difficulties initially because the coalition consisted largely of individuals who worked with intervention services and did not have the time or interest to work with prevention. She also had difficulty adjusting to the shift from direct services to prevention. A new program coordinator committed to prevention worked with the local coalition (CCR) to modify the composition of the committee and develop a mission statement focused on prevention of IPV and SV. The coalition wished to identify current risks and protective factors for being a victim or a perpetrator, including the examination of attitudes, beliefs, and behaviors of adolescents and adults that promoted or endorsed SV, and to develop partnerships and collaborations to develop a comprehensive program to reduce victimization or perpetration. Because young adult males who score high on rape-myth acceptance measures and believe relationships are adversarial are also more likely to report having committed rape

(Loh, Gidycz, Lobo, & Luthra, 2005), the coalition focused on learning more about attitudes through surveys and focus groups.

Description of process for conducting needs and resource assessment: method

After reviewing the literature regarding attitudes as a risk factor for IPV and SV, the coalition conducted a randomized telephone survey of adults in their community, followed by a number of focus groups of middle, high, and vocational school students and undergraduate students. The empowerment evaluators provided assistance in data collection and analysis and recruited a research center to complete the randomized telephone survey.

Example of results

The community attitude survey found that males, $t(355) = 2.49$, $p = .013$, lower income respondents, $F(4, 280) = 9.70$, $p = .000$, and persons whose highest degree was high school, $F(3, 326) = 4.69$, $p = .003$, held the most traditional gender norms. Focus groups revealed attitudes among some adolescents supportive of SV, such as the belief that consent for sexual activity was required if one was dating another person but not if he or she were "hooking up" and that, if someone dressed in a certain way, he or she was "asking" to be sexually active or sexually assaulted. In addition to the results of the survey and focus groups, community attitudes were apparent through the process of data collection. Men were more likely to refuse to participate than females when called regarding the survey, and the refusal rate of males was higher than is typical for phone surveys. A state legislator was disgruntled with the agency for conducting the survey. The school system would not allow the CCR to survey students in the school system. There was also some hesitancy in the community to address issues of sexual objectification of women, as evidenced by resistance in the community to an awareness campaign regarding billboard advertizing that objectified women. This led to a lively debate in the community about SV issues but also led to the loss of one committee member whose agency felt they could no longer participate in this prevention program. In addition the RACC lost a large private donation due to negative community reaction to efforts to prevent IPV and SV.

Factors That Contributed to the Success of the Projects

Success was considered to be the completion of a N&R assessment that reflected the local community and provided support for the development of a local plan to prevent IPV and SV. One author representing a local program stated, though, that true success would be "when the plan is accepted, embraced, implemented, and we can see changes being made in the attitudes of the boys now who will be young men in 5 to 8 years." Common individual, organizational, and community factors contributed to the success of the projects.

Individual staff implementing the projects

In each of the three communities, staff implementing the project brought individual strengths, including experience in the field of IPV and SV, flexibility, and the ability to think critically. The need for flexibility was characterized by one woman's comment, "learning from mistakes and changing directions when necessary." They were truly generalist practitioners, working with individual clients in crisis, collaborating with other organizations, and participating in media events. As providers of direct services to victims, they stated that they initially felt out of their element in the role of practitioner/researcher. In spite of this, they agreed to participate in a program with (1) an external conceptual framework and structure provided by the CDC, (2) a requirement for participation in ongoing technical assistance that included group trainings in a central location and onsite consultation by state level project staff and evaluators, (3) the expectation that other community partners would be engaged in the project, and (4) the obligation for completion of a local N&R assessment.

Each of the three programs requested technical assistance regarding the N&R assessment and participated actively in the process. They used theory to guide their work and visualized complex data collection procedures and participated in data collection, analysis, and dissemination. In one case, the staff person thought that her academic preparation in the sciences stood her in good stead in conceptualizing and implementing their project and writing their report. Staff turnover was limited. One staff stated that their success was as a result of taking "one step at a time." This ability to partialize may be critical in the successful implementation of such a complex program.

Organizational context

Each local program supported the project and project staff. The director of one organization, who sat on the state-level prevention coalition, provided the prevention staff member "tethered freedom" to do the prevention work. Another director attended all the technical assistance meetings with the staff person implementing this project.

Community coalitions

In each community, the local coalition played a key role in the development of the project. Leaders emerged in each community. Coalition members' participation may have occurred outside formal meetings and ranged from providing access to the school setting for data collection to assisting with data analysis.

Broader environmental factors, including the state and national project

EMPOWER and DELTA staff working for the CDC provided extensive technical assistance, in addition to funding. Technical assistance included information regarding the initial model to be implemented, written resources including research articles, face-to-face grantee meetings, phone conferences, and site visits. The state program staff and empowerment evaluators provided extensive technical assistance to local communities, passing information along from the national technical assistance opportunities. In addition to the face-to-face meetings (group trainings and site visits), phone conferences, and e-mail communications, the project used Blackboard, a Website for sharing documents. State staff and the evaluators were able to link local staff to other resources, also, such as other local community members and organizations and to data collection support such as the University of North Dakota Social Science Research Institute, who provided valuable expertise and resources.

Conceptual framework

The national project had a well-defined conceptual framework. Each local community identified a conceptual framework specific to their community and project that was congruent with the overarching conceptual framework.

Challenges

The three communities experienced several challenges, from the individual to broader societal issues. One staff member summarized the challenges to completing the N&R assessment:

> Challenges were getting men who were willing to share why they aren't sex offenders. Getting people to talk about it, and then maintaining the team, the energy, the focus, how to get people to hang their hats on this important issue when there are so many out there pining for their attention. Taking so much information and narrowing it down to focus on where the most good can be done with limited resources.

Challenges occurred with the conceptualization of the project, state-level support, and community issues.

Conceptual framework

The GTO process was being developed throughout the project, which meant that national- and state-level staff were learning just ahead of the local entities.

Individuals and local organizations implementing prevention programs

The public health approach and prevention principles were new for organizations that traditionally provided direct services to victims of IPV and SV, their community coalitions, and many others statewide. One staff person said she was initially "taken aback" by the project.

Community coalitions

In each community, coalitions focusing on prevention of IPV and SV were a new concept, requiring development of new partnerships. Persons participating in coalitions were busy and had difficulty finding time to attend meetings, despite their interest. The level of community readiness varied within communities, leading to conflict between people and organizations regarding prevention of IPV and SV.

Broader environmental factors, including the state and national project

The entire original staff at the state level, including the funding agency, the state-level organization directing the project, and the evaluation team, changed during the project period. Funding was limited, especially for programs doing only SV prevention.

DISCUSSION

Summary of Key Findings

This project demonstrated that communities can successfully implement complex programs, in spite of initial trepidation and lack of previous experience with the public health approach, GTO, and empowerment evaluation. Developing a N&R assessment using the empowerment evaluation and GTO process was intensive, requiring a great deal of stamina and persistence on the part of all involved, and these three programs demonstrated they were up to the challenge. Successful implementation occurred when the model addressed multiple systems levels, involved persons it targeted in its development, and provided opportunities for individualizing at the local level. The prevention of IPV and SV project incorporated intensive technical assistance at the local, state, and national levels.

Lessons Learned

Conceptual framework

Feminist theory, as described in the integrative feminist model (McPhail, Busch, Kulkarni, & Rice, 2007), empowerment evaluation, and family social work theory have common tenets that can be integrated to support prevention of IPV and SV. Empowerment evaluation, a strengths-based model focusing on agencies' and individuals' ability to become more competent in conducting and using evaluation, emphasizes the ability of individuals and/or organizations to grow and become self-evaluating. Empowerment evaluation rejects the traditional adversarial role between the evaluator and those being evaluated and emphasizes partnerships between the empowerment evaluator and program staff. Empowerment evaluation, with its emphasis on democratic participation and social justice, values input from all stakeholders in the design and implementation of evaluation. Feminist theory, the undergirding of the domestic violence movement which began in the 1970s, addresses power and procedures for changing power, as does empowerment evaluation (Frisby, Maguire, & Reid, 2009) and family social work (McPhail et al., 2007; National Association of Social Workers [NASW], 2008). The integrative feminist model, like empowerment evaluation's value for social justice, "hold[s] tightly to the strengths of the feminist model that acknowledges the political and social structures that perpetuate inequality such as the unequal distribution of resources on the basis of gender, race, class, sexual orientation, age, and disability" (McPhail et al., 2007, p. 838).

Individuals, organizations, and communities prevention of intimate partner and sexual violence

The three programs were successful in part because women implementing the prevention project were from the area where the projects emerged. Because the women were "locals," they understood how to focus their community efforts toward prevention that would be acceptable in their area. Although the women doing local prevention programming saw themselves as being out of their element initially, they identified the empowerment evaluator as the catalyst for change. Women who were successfully intervening in IPV and SV situations became successful at prevention activities, also. Individuals implementing the project had to have multiple abilities, from interpersonal relationships to writing to thinking critically to flexibility and persistence. One commented: "This was a project that required an investment of the heart—you had to strongly believe in what you were doing and be able to see the big picture and the results that could be achieved not only in the near future but also down the road."

Broader environmental factors influencing prevention efforts

Technical assistance by empowerment evaluators was a critical component for successful completion of the N&R assessment. Understanding a local community's level of readiness for change was also essential in completing the N&R assessment and moving forward with planning for prevention of IPV and SV.

Strengths and Limitations of Study

The strengths and limitations of the method for this project are related. Because the authors were intimately involved with the development of the project, they have extensive knowledge about it. They also therefore are biased; the stories and the analysis of those stories reflect the multiple perspectives of local staff developing and implementing the project, community coalition members, and empowerment evaluators. The results may not be generalizable to other communities who have different individual, geographic, population, and political characteristics.

Implications of Study and Recommendations

Taking the lessons learned from this project and applying them in different communities will further inform the question about what impact the empowerment evaluation process has on developing successful prevention programs. Creating a standardized method for evaluating outcomes and the processes that led to those outcomes will allow comparison across many similar projects and further inform the generalizability of results. Following the progress of these three communities will provide information about the long-term impact of applying empowerment evaluation principles to prevention of IPV and SV in local communities.

Local programs identified critical areas for working with families that can inform the efforts of family social workers. Early childhood events within the family were identified as contributing to perpetration. Family social workers can contribute to prevention of IPV and SV in many ways:

1. developing parenting models that increase positive parenting (to prevent IPV and SV focusing on families
2. addressing situational couple violence (Johnson & Leone, 2005)
3. implementing early intervention programs designed to prevent child abuse and neglect (Arndt & Horodynski, 2004)
4. serving as empowerment evaluators.

REFERENCES

Arndt, M. J., & Horodynski, M. A. (2004). Theory of dependent-care in research with parents of toddlers: The NEAT Project. *Nursing Science Quarterly*, *17*, 345–350.

Basile, K. C., Espelage, D. L., Rivers, I., McMahon, P. M., & Simon, T. R. (2009). The theoretical and empirical links between bullying behavior and male sexual violence perpetration. *Aggression and Violent Behavior*, *14*(5), 336–347.

Bohner, G., Siebler, F., & Schmelcher, J. (2006). Social norms and the likelihood of raping: Perceived rape myth acceptance of others affects men's rape proclivity. *Personality and Social Psychology Bulletin, 32*(3), 286–297.

Bordeaux, B. C., Wiley, C., Tandon, D., Horowitz, C. R., Bohrer Brown, P., & Bass, E. B. (2007). Guidelines for writing manuscripts about community-based participatory research for peer-reviewed journals. *The Johns Hopkins University Press, 1*(3), 281–288.

Bronfenbrenner, U., & Ceci, S. J. (1994). Nature-nurture reconceptualized in developmental perspective: A bioecological model. *Psychological Review, 101*(4), 568–586.

Chinman, M., Imm, P., & Wandersman, A. (2004). *Getting to Outcomes 2004: Promoting accountability through methods and tools for planning, implementation, and evaluation.* Santa Monica, CA: RAND Corporation.

Coulter, M. (2004). *The impact of domestic violence on the employment of women on welfare.* Washington, DC: U.S. Department of Justice.

Cox, P., Ortega, S., Cook-Craig, P. G., & Conway, P. (2010). Strengthening systems for the primary prevention of sexual violence and intimate partner violence: CDC's DELTA and EMPOWER programs. *Journal of Family Social Work, 13*(4), 287–296.

Daeg de Mott, D. K. (2009, May 18). Kohlberg's theory of moral reasoning. *Encyclopedia of Childhood and Adolescence.* Retrieved from http://findarticles.com/p/articles/mi_g2602/is_0003/ai_2602000337/

Fetterman, D., Kaftarian, S. J., & Wandersman, A. (1995). Empowerment evaluation: Knowledge and tools for self-assessment and accountability.

Fetterman, D. M., & Wandersman, A. (Eds.). (2005). *Empowerment evaluation principles in practice.* New York: Guilford.

Frisby, W., Maguire, P., & Reid, C. (2009). The 'f' word has everything to do with it: How feminist theories inform action research. *Action Research, 7*, 13–29.

Gilgun, J. F., Daly, K., & Handel, G. (Eds.). (1992). *Qualitative methods in family research.* Newbury Park, CA: Sage.

Glaser, B., & Strauss, A. (1967). *The discovery of grounded theory. Strategies for qualitative research.* Chicago: Aldine Publishing Co.

Johnson, M. P., & Leone, J. M. (2005). The differential effects of intimate terrorism and situational couple violence. *Journal of Family Issues, 26*, 322–349.

Loh, C., Gidycz, C. A., Lobo, T. R., & Luthra, R. (2005). A prospective analysis of sexual assault perpetration: Risk factors related to perpetrator characteristics. *Journal of Interpersonal Violence, 20*, 1325–1348.

McPhail, B. A., Busch, N. B., Kulkarni, S., & Rice, G. (2007). An integrative feminist model: The evolving feminist perspective on intimate partner violence. *Violence Against Women, 13*, 817–840.

Miller, R. L., & Campbell, R. (2006). Taking stock of empowerment evaluation. *American Journal of Evaluation, 27*(3), 296–319.

National Association of Social Workers. (2008). *NASW Code of Ethics.* Retrieved from http://www.naswdc.org/pubs/code/code.asp

National Center for Injury Prevention and Control. (2002). *CDC injury research agenda.* Atlanta, GA: Centers for Disease Control and Prevention.

Olweis, D. (1993). *Bullying at school.* Malden, MA: Blackwell Publishing.

Steckler, A., & Linnan, L. (Eds.). (2002). *Process evaluation for public health interventions and research*. San Francisco: Jossey-Bass.

Tjaden, P., & Thoennes, N. (1998). *Prevalence, incidence, and consequences of violence against women: Findings from the national violence against women survey*. National Institute of Justice Centers for Disease Control and Prevention.

University of North Dakota, School of Medicine and Health Sciences, Department of Community Medicine. (2004, August). *Behavioral risks reported by American Indian adults in North Dakota: 1996–2002*. Bismarck, ND: North Dakota Department of Health.

U.S. Census Bureau. (2009). *State and county quick facts*. Retrieved from http://quickfacts.census.gov/qfd/states/38000.html

Yin, R. K. (2003). *Case study research: Design and methods* (3rd ed.). Thousand Oaks, CA: Sage.

Youth Action Strategies in the Primary Prevention of Teen Dating Violence

DENISE KERVIN
Family Support Center, Chippewa Falls, Wisconsin

JENNIFER OBINNA
World Bridge Research, Minnetonka, Minnesota

This article describes a school-based youth-driven teen dating violence prevention project. The project objectives are to provide opportunities for students to plan presentations and activities; develop knowledge and awareness about unhealthy gender norms, seen as an important root cause of relationship violence, particularly for teenagers; and identify ways to cope with and influence their environment with respect to this issue. This project was conducted in a rural Wisconsin community over the course of 5 years. It started as a multischool "drop-in" program with students from various high schools but eventually evolved into a youth action team at an alternative high school as a for-credit service learning class. Evaluation findings show the project to have promise in changing individual attitudes and beliefs while promoting bystander intervention. This youth-led health approach provides excellent opportunities for youth to become involved and empowered, and collaborating with schools can also be a successful strategy. Because unhealthy gender norms are so deeply entrenched, it is important to document and celebrate the smallest positive shifts in attitudes and behaviors.

Dating violence is commonly suggested to be a type of intimate partner violence (IPV) occurring between two people in a close relationship. The nature of dating violence can be physical, emotional, or sexual (Centers for Disease Control & Prevention [CDC], 2009). Teen dating violence is a serious problem, with estimates of physical and sexual dating violence among high school students ranging from 10% to 25% (Silverman, Raj, Mucci, & Hathaway, 2001; Wekerle & Wolfe, 1999), and even higher estimates are found when verbal threats and emotional abuse are considered (Jezl, Molidor, & Wright, 1996).

To construct a community-specific teen dating violence prevention program in rural Wisconsin, local family support workers, social service agencies, and representatives from the criminal justice system conducted a needs assessment to identify risk, protective, and causal factors that should be addressed. To complete this needs assessment four focus groups were held with teens, professionals, parents, and lesbian, gay, bisexual, and transgendered youth. Risk factors that emerged included (1) ongoing family violence, (2) economic problems, (3) mental health issues, and (4) unhealthy gender norms. All four focus groups identified the importance of gender stereotypes, such as that a male has the right or "duty" to be the controlling partner, or that a female's worth is largely determined by having and keeping a male partner.

According to a World Health Organization report, males who hold traditional gender norms have a higher likelihood of committing IPV (Heise & Garcia-Moreno, 2002). It is also suggested that "sexual violence occurs in part due to peer support for sexually adversarial attitudes and behaviors amongst groups of men" (Brown et al., n.d.).

Building on the notion that unhealthy gender norms are an important risk factor associated with teen dating violence, the health belief model (HBM) has been identified as a possible approach for primary prevention programs (Aiken, Gerend, & Jackson, 2001). The HBM is an extensively studied model of health behavior change that suggests that individuals who perceive themselves at risk for a health threat will take actions to reduce risky behaviors or to engage in healthy alternative behaviors. Donna Garske, with Transforming Communities, argued that gender norms support individuals' knowledge-attitudes-beliefs-behaviors (KABBs), including those related to relationships (Garske, 2004). Garske suggested that changing unhealthy gender norms will reduce the risk of unhealthy relationships and teen dating violence.

DESCRIPTION OF THE PROGRAM

Two types of youth action strategies are most commonly cited in the literature. The first focuses upon social action and civic engagement where service learning opportunities and volunteering in a range of organizations is employed. This is done primarily to enhance the individual youth's experience in the world while assisting people in need or building community. The second has been called transformational youth action because it strives to alter the social conditions in a community that perpetuate a social problem. This transformational approach challenges the status quo and is concerned with changing political structures (Morsillo & Prilleltensky, 2007). Borrowing in part from both types of youth action strategies, the Youth Advisory Committee (YAC), in the rural Wisconsin county of Chippewa, was born.

Background

The YAC began during the 2004–2005 school year, with the goal of working to prevent teen dating violence through the collaboration of high school students across the county. The YAC met in the evenings and weekends; and, not surprisingly, the meetings were often poorly attended, impeding setting goals for the group and gaining momentum. In considering solutions, the program designers were influenced by the importance of "saturating" versus "sprinkling," which the Southern California Injury Prevention Research Center (2008) eloquently described:

> Addressing the most relevant risk and resilience factors and doing so in a way that will have the intended impact within identified neighborhoods, communities, schools, or cities requires bringing programs, practices, and policies to scale with adequate *staffing, training*, and *funding*. Too often, efforts are scattered, and precious resources are dissipated. Over time, it is critical to have enough saturation of programs, practices, and policies to have an impact on an identified population (e.g., a specific neighborhood, 14–19 year olds, etc.) and to be able to bring that investment to scale so outcomes can be sustained and violence will be prevented, rather than simply displaced to another location. (p. 4)

In 2005 and 2006 the YAC moved to the alternative high school, Chippewa Valley High School (CVHS), as an after-school program. Holding the group with just one school's students as members meant shifting from an attempt to influence as many youth as possible—a "sprinkling" approach—to focusing on "saturating" that smaller group of teens for a more profound and longer-lasting impact.

Entry into the YAC was controlled; students were invited to join by CVHS's social worker. Students who rejected relationship violence and seemed to be potential positive role models for healthy relationships were invited to join. Attendance stayed fairly steady over the school years, with about 10 to 12 students beginning each year and about 4 to 8 at the end. This attrition stemmed from students graduating at midyear, returning to their regular school, or dropping out of school entirely. A few students were asked to leave the group because they used violence or relied on sexist gender norms. The students then changed the name from the Youth Advisory

Committee to the Youth Action Committee, signaling their desire to actively prevent teen dating violence by creating and delivering presentations to other teens and adults.

In 2007 the YAC transformed into a high school for-credit service learning class geared toward learning about and working to prevent IPV in youth. The process of moving the YAC from a more informal group to a for-credit class relied on guidelines delineated in the document *Principles of Effective Prevention Programs* (Nation et al., 2003; see Table 1).

The class was cotaught twice a week by the Domestic Violence Prevention Enhancements and Leadership Through Alliances (DELTA) coordinator

TABLE 1 Prevention Principles and Application in Youth Advisory Committee (YAC) Class

Prevention principles	YAC class
Appropriately timed: Does the program come at an appropriate point in the participant's development and ability to change?	The students in YAC have often experienced IPV and feel strongly about preventing it in their and others' lives, so the timing is ideal. They are also young enough to have a better chance of changing unhealthy attitudes and behaviors compared with an adult.
Sufficient dosage: Is there adequate exposure to the program's material?	Turning YAC into a class meant working with the students over an entire school year, meeting for 50 minutes twice a week for 9 months.
Comprehensive: Do the program strategies include multiple components and affect multiple settings to address a wide range of risk and protective factors?	The YAC class and student-created presentations address unhealthy gender norms and youth leadership development as a comprehensive strategy of building self-esteem while enhancing student change with a "learning while teaching" approach.
Positive relationships: Are strong relationships fostered between adults and youth?	The class has two coteachers, plus undergraduate interns, who work on establishing positive and supportive relationships with YAC members each year. One of the coteachers is the school social worker who interacts with YAC members daily in that capacity.
Theory based: Is the program based on theories shown to lead to change?	The Project draws on theories about gender ideology and creating change through addressing the health beliefs model of changing knowledge, attitudes, beliefs and behaviors.
Varied teaching methods: does the program use different methods, addressing different learning styles?	The YAC class uses different teaching methods, including discussion, lecture, activities, and media to address the students' learning styles. In addition, students often attend conferences to broaden their knowledge and experiences.

and CVHS social worker, usually with the assistance of undergraduate social work interns from nearby universities. The first semester focuses on the knowledge, attitudes, beliefs, and behaviors underlying unhealthy and healthy relationships, and the role of gender norms in relationship violence. Constructivist learning theory suggests that one of the best ways to learn and retain information and skills is to teach about them (Brooks & Brooks, 1993), therefore the YAC spends the second semester designing and giving presentations, primarily to middle schoolers in the county. The class also works within CVHS all year to raise awareness of teen dating violence and the qualities of healthy relationships. Although this approach has had many successes, the project also has faced many challenges along the design journey, particularly learning the public health approach and planning strategies, as well as working with teens in an alternative high school.

Learning the Public Health Approach

In 2003 the Wisconsin Coalition Against Domestic Violence (WCADV) learned that the CDC was interested in demonstrating new and innovative programs that focused on the primary prevention of IPV. The CDC's new program was called DELTA. These "alliances" were local coalitions that the CDC was interested in working with, called coordinated community response coalitions (CCRs). CCRs work to improve the systems involved with domestic violence and sexual assault victims and perpetrators, including criminal justice and victim services. Members are largely involved in the intervention of IPV; one aspect of the DELTA project was to test whether CCRs can also incorporate a primary prevention focus: can they respond to existing IPV and try to address its risk and protective factors in order to prevent it.

After being awarded DELTA funding by the CDC, WCADV invited communities across Wisconsin to submit proposals for projects focused on the primary prevention of IPV. Chippewa County's CCR had a strong history of interest in prevention, particularly for a youth population. Although very interested in promoting prevention of teen dating violence, the CCR was challenged by the learning involved in creating this project. For many members, thinking in terms of primary prevention meant putting aside their daily intervention mind-set and learning new mind-sets like the public health approach. Throughout the early years of the project, CCR members attended trainings held by WCADV and the DELTA coordinator focused on the differences between primary prevention and intervention strategies.

In 2007 a survey was conducted in which CCR members ($N=6$) were asked whether scenarios described primary prevention strategies. Although most members answered with the desirable response on 6 of the 8 scenarios, 67% (4) of the members thought that holding a candlelight vigil to raise awareness was a primary prevention activity. Candlelight vigils focus on supporting survivorship and do not seek to stop root causes, such as unhealthy gender norms. Also, 50% (3) mistakenly thought that training clergy to recognize the signs of abuse was also a primary prevention activity. Because of the results from this survey, further discussion was held with CCR members to clarify the differences between primary prevention and intervention.

Working With Teens in an Alternative High School

Besides the challenges faced in learning the public health approach and moving from an intervention to a primary prevention mind-set, the program' designers had to discover how to best work with the alternative high school. In many ways, this school is the ideal location for YAC as many of the students have experienced the causal and risk factors identified in the focus groups, such as witnessing domestic violence in their homes or having economic problems. The school is also flexible in dealing with the students, allowing them to travel outside the building for presentations and to go to conferences.

On the other hand, students attend the alternative school because they are in danger of not graduating. Often this situation arises from mental health issues, such as depression or anxiety, substance abuse issues, or learning difficulties, such as attention deficit/hyperactivity disorder. Thus, many YAC members are easily distracted, have trouble focusing on the task at hand, and need different types of support to learn. In addition, many of the students have chaotic home lives, causing them to miss class or be inattentive when present. One strategy used to address some of these problems involves activities that address different learning styles, such as information sheets about healthy relationship skills paired with skits in which students practice these skills through acting. Another strategy is having "toys," such as squishy balls, for students to handle to allow them to more easily focus on class topics. It is beneficial that one of the YAC's coteachers is the school's social worker and so knows what is happening in each student's life and can interact with each appropriately.

EVALUATION

A pre- and posttest to measure the impact of YAC on its members was developed by identifying unhealthy gender norms and identifying the relevant knowledge, attitudes, beliefs, and behaviors that could be addressed in developing teens. The YAC pretest is administered within the first 2 weeks of class, then at the end of the school year, or when students leave YAC. Attrition from students graduating, leaving school, or being dropped from YAC is a concern. Approximately 25% to 50% of the class will have left the class by the end of the year; however, before these students leave they are asked to complete the posttest.

Besides pre- and posttests, other data is gathered from YAC members using a variety of qualitative sources. The students do written activities in class that offer insight into their gender beliefs, including a survey on gender norms that is repeated at the end of the year. Observational data from discussions during the YAC class and other classes at CVHS is also documented.

Pre- and Posttest Results

Pretest data exists for 48 students, along with posttest data for 29 students, over the course of four school years (see Tables 2–4). Inferential statistics were not used to analyze this data. Practitioner-driven programs sometimes have difficulty compiling and analyzing data. In the past, staff often read through or "eye-balled" data. For this project efforts were made to enter data into Microsoft Excel for analysis using descriptive statistics. This modest modification in data entry and analysis allowed program designers to have more information than before about what was occurring with the program participants and where to focus future project changes. It is also a sustainable data management evaluation strategy that can be maintained over time.

One goal of the YAC class was to lessen the likelihood that members would use abusive behaviors, such as physical violence, within their relationships. It should be noted that, for this set of questions, the students in YAC started with high percentages of desirable answers; most initial responses were in the 80% to 90% range (see Table 2). This may be due in large part to the fact that students were carefully chosen to have an interest in preventing teen dating violence and displaying behavior that suggests they would be good role models.

TABLE 2 Descriptive Comparison of Desirable Responses: Avoiding Physical Abuse

Would you "Probably Not" or "Definitely Not" be likely to do something like hit or push your boyfriend/girlfriend if he/she:	Pretest		Posttest	
	n	%	*n*	%
Called you nasty names	41	85	23	79
Wouldn't leave you alone	42	88	26	90
Yelled at you	38	79	24	83
Followed you around when you said not to	44	92	24	83
Ignored you	44	92	26	90
Flirted with your best friend	33	69	19	66
Put you down in front of your friends	37	77	21	72
Hit or pushed you	24	50	16	55
Broke up with you	46	96	28	97
Wouldn't shut up	41	85	26	90

Note: Pretest $N = 48$, Posttest = 29.

It is impossible to determine without the use of inferential statistics whether some of these changes from the pretest to the posttest are significant. The students' responses were helpful in highlighting areas requiring additional attention in class. The teens particularly struggled with partners who were flirtatious, verbally or physically abusive (see Table 2). Because of the low scores on both the pre- and post-tests, more class time will be devoted to these areas.

Another set of pre- and post-test questions examined the students' likelihood of engaging in healthy relationship behaviors, such as communicating about their feelings and controlling their anger (see Table 3). The YAC class included discussions about these positive behaviors, many of which became the focus of the skits performed by the YAC. Without inferential statistics it is impossible to determine if the increases in most items from pre-tests to post-tests is significant. However, the numbers indicated the need to address students' handling of criticism, anger and jealousy.

A final set of pre- and post-test questions examined students' gender norms and bystander skills (see Table 4). Because unhealthy gender norms were seen as an important root cause of teen dating violence, much time was spent examining assumptions about masculinity and femininity in the YAC class. The goal was to encourage YAC members to consider and possibly change their own gender beliefs and related behaviors. An additional goal of the YAC class was to increase appropriate "bystander skills," that is, responding when another person is speaking in a sexist or violent way. The movement of student answers from pre- to post-tests was in the desired direction, especially regarding whether they would react to another person's inappropriate behaviors. During class and in the YAC's presentations, there was a focus on when and how to "call" someone on behavior supporting unhealthy gender norms. For example, many of the YAC's presentations over the years included a skit in which a male was being put down because he

TABLE 3 Descriptive Comparison of Desirable Responses: Relationship Interaction

	Pretest		Posttest	
With your boyfriend/girlfriend are you "Likely" or "Very Likely" to:	*n*	%	*n*	%
Deal with serious disagreements honestly & directly	39	81	25	86
Openly talk about what you want	39	81	27	93
Say when you feel hurt/upset with his or her opinions	38	79	23	79
Show respect when you disagree with his or her opinions	40	83	26	90
Control your temper when she or he is angry with you	36	75	23	79
Accept reasonable criticism from him or her without getting really upset	32	67	22	76
Control your temper when you are angry	32	67	23	79
Control feelings of jealousy	29	60	17	59
Work out minor problems together	44	92	26	90

Note: Pretest $N = 48$, Posttest $= 29$.

TABLE 4 Descriptive Comparison of Desirable Responses: Gender Assumptions and Bystander Behavior

	Pretest		Posttest	
I agree with the following statements:	*n*	%	*n*	%
I believe that talking with a new boyfriend/girlfriend about expectations of our relationship destroys romance.	29	60	18	62
A male can control his behavior no matter how angry or sexually aroused he is.	35	73	26	90
I believe that alcohol affects my decisions and actions.	30	63	18	62
When a female says "no" to physical affection or sex, it never means "maybe."	44	92	27	93
If you heard someone you know putting females down, you would ask them to stop.	41	85	27	93
You don't listen to music with lyrics that are violent/disrespectful to women.	11	23	7	24
If you heard someone you know putting males down, you would ask them to stop.	30	63	22	76
If you see a guy you know saying something to a female and you know she doesn't like it, you would ask him to stop.	37	77	27	93
If you see a guy you don't know saying something to a female, and you know she doesn't like it you ask him to stop.	30	63	24	83

Note: Pretest $N=48$, Posttest $=29$.

wasn't good at sports. The role playing showed how to respond to such behavior in a nonviolent way, as the person being bullied and as a bystander.

Given the importance of popular culture's role in supporting unhealthy relationships and violence in general, the students' lack of change from pretest to posttest responses (23% to 24%) to "You don't listen to music with lyrics that are violent/disrespectful to women" was disappointing. The YAC students had trouble seeing the connection between listening to music with sexist or violent lyrics and supporting the continuation of relationship violence. Because of how entrenched this behavior seems, and the teens' beliefs that such personal action has no larger societal impact, more class time was devoted to the topic.

Qualitative Results

In-class written activities and observations from discussions offered insight into students' gender beliefs. Observations and self-reports indicated that most YAC members attempted to incorporate skills from class into their ongoing relationships. For example, one former YAC student shared at a reunion in 2008: "Since being a YAC member, I try to use what I have learned to create more healthy relationships in my life.... If I am in a confrontation with someone or trying to talk to a friend I think about the things we presented in YAC to effectively get my point across." Another student at the end of the 2007–2008 school year stated in a written evaluation: "I have learned a lot about different types of [healthy and unhealthy] behaviors. I look at what people are doing and think 'That's not good behavior.' Also I think I learned a better outlook on life."

One of YAC's coteachers, in her role as the school's social worker, saw the YAC students' behaviors changing across the school year. For example, she indicated that physical violence decreased and students began to react negatively to sexist jokes, such as by not laughing or by walking away. Sometimes students indicated that YAC had a profound impact on their lives. At the aforementioned reunion a former YAC member wrote: "The knowledge helped a lot. My thinking and behavior went from angry and violent to caring and realizing that many situations were wrong in my life. You saved me from what could've been years of destroying behavior."

Unintended Successes

It also appears that being part of YAC has helped many students work on changing their KABBs outside of school. Every year YAC members are encouraged to identify their attitudes and/or behaviors that reinforce unhealthy gender norms and work on changing one or two, with the support of other members. Outside of class these students therefore contribute to a more "saturated" environment as they remind one another of the changes they are trying to make in themselves. This is often very important as many students who become YAC members will still remain friends with students who hold unhealthy KABBs.

YAC has also been beneficial to CVHS by bringing in additional adults to work with their students and offering YAC students new opportunities, such as doing presentations and going to conferences. An unforeseen benefit for the high school is that the YAC combats widely-held assumptions about alternative school students: that they are troublemakers, lazy, and unintelligent. It has been a source of pride for YAC groups to change community members' minds and improve the reputation of the alternative high school.

Finally, it was a significant success to have YAC become a for-credit service learning class at the alternative high school. First, such a status ensures its sustainability. Second, though many schools incorporate prevention lessons and even units into their curriculum, much more change can be accomplished in a regularly-meeting, two-semester class. The YAC class also offers a model for other schools and organizations interested in primary prevention of IPV in teens.

Lessons Learned

During the 3rd year, the program designers conducted a process evaluation, using interviews and document reviews, which pointed to reasons the YAC ran successfully. An important finding was that it is imperative to have a group like the YAC housed in a stable setting, such as a school. Potentially, a church youth group or even a setting such as a Boys and Girls Club could work, as long as youth can meet there regularly. It was also determined that it is necessary to have the full support of the site sponsoring such a group, with a key collaborator in that setting serving as a liaison between the staff and the fiscal agent. For this project it was the social worker at the alternative high school.

In conjunction with a stable setting, running a group like the YAC requires that the meetings fit into everyone's schedules. Because of interest generated at a YAC presentation given in 2005 to groups of high school students from around the county, a YAC group was begun at another high school in the county. This was a smaller group of students who had to meet before or after their school day. An AmeriCorps volunteer helped to coordinate that group, as well as the teens at the alternative high school. Although there was success in that both YAC groups did presentations for their communities that school year, doing the second YAC project in the new high school became logistically more and more difficult, and thus this strategy was dropped.

Students seem to work best when they feel ownership of the group, such as through making planning decisions and seeing their work appreciated by others, especially during presentations. Although putting a measure of control in the YAC members' hands was difficult because of the real potential for missteps, the coteachers felt that mistakes are part of the learning process. It is also important that fun be mixed in regularly with learning and preparing for presentations. YAC members often enter or stay in the group because they have friends in the class.

Students also demand to see their reality acknowledged, which in the YAC includes acknowledging that males are abused by females. Male and female students are adamant that they know young men being emotionally, verbally, and even physically abused by girlfriends. From class discussions, it seems that such abuse is vastly underreported, in part because of the gender norms maintaining that males should be able to deal with violence and should not ask for help.

Besides learning about practical considerations in running a YAC class, realistic expectations in creating change in teens were also learned. During a meeting at the end of the 2008–2009 school year, the CVHS school social worker stated: "We want to see big results," but acknowledged that such a desire may set the project up for failure. Ideally, students would leave YAC with healthy attitudes about gender norms and relationships, with behaviors to match, and a desire to change their peers' unhealthy KABBs. However, realistically, primary prevention projects have to be content with making a small, but real, difference in the lives of students.

The YAC coteachers believe that the changes made by YAC members are in large part due to the intensity of the project. The YAC is definitely a "saturation," not a "sprinkling," strategy. A small group of teens are engaged across an entire school year, forging close relationships and building trust with each other and with caring adults. The resulting rapport helps the students more readily embrace the changes being encouraged in their KABBs.

The relationships formed in YAC frequently continue after graduation. Often former YAC members will visit after graduating, seeking out the social worker and talking about the impact of YAC. The connections made in the group also seem to help students maintain changes to their KABBs after graduating. Feedback from the 2008 reunion suggested that former YAC members who continued to spend time together had more behaviors consistent with the class than those without such contact. Thus, maintaining YAC friendships seems to provide necessary support for healthy KABBs, even as they are challenged by new acquaintances and society in general.

CONCLUSION

Primary prevention work takes optimism and patience. Seeing what a tenacious hold IPV's root causes have on society and individuals, it is easy to become discouraged when trying to create change. The YAC has provided insight into realistic expectations and helpful tools to try to reach project goals. Ideally, a primary prevention program for youth needs a stable home and the means to be sustainable. Collaborating with a school can be a successful approach. A program also needs a foundation of knowledge about how to create social change and a structure that appeals to and obtains buy-in from its participants. Last, program staff and participants should notice and celebrate baby steps in IPV prevention and shifting social norms. When a student stops herself from saying a habitual gendered put-down, or a male explains to a group of younger students that his acting the "big, tough guy" role in the past only brought him grief, it is a significant step for the youth and a small—but important—shift toward a world free of dating violence.

REFERENCES

Aiken, L. S., Gerend, M. A., & Jackson, K. M. (2001). Subjective risk and health protective behavior: Cancer screening and cancer prevention. In A. Baum, T. A. Revenson, & J. E. Singer (Eds.), *Handbook of health psychology* (pp. 727–746). Mahwah, NJ: Erlbaum Associates.

Brooks, J., & Brooks, M. (1993). *In search of understanding: The case for constructivist classrooms.* Alexandria, VA: Association for Supervision & Curriculum Development.

Brown, P., Cascone, L., Flowers, J., Foster, H., Furrow, A., Hart, C., et al. (n.d.). *Guidelines for the primary prevention of sexual violence & intimate partner violence.* Richmond, VA: Virginia Sexual & Domestic Violence Action Alliance.

Centers for Disease Control and Prevention. (2009). *Teen dating violence fact sheet.* Atlanta GA: CDC, National Center for Injury Prevention and Control.

Garske, D. (2004, August 12). *Mobilizing the community for domestic violence prevention.* Poster session presented at the WCADV DELTA Conference, Madison, Wisconsin.

Heise, L., & Garcia-Moreno, C. (2002). Violence by intimate partners. In E. Krug, L. Dahlberg, J. Mercy, A. Zwi, & R. Loran. (Eds.), *World report on violence and health* (pp. 87–122). Geneva, Switzerland: World Health Organization.

Jezl, D. R., Molidor, C. E., & Wright, T. L. (1996). Physical, sexual, and psychological abuse in high school dating relationships: Prevalence rates and self-esteem issues. *Child and Adolescent Social Work Journal, 13*(1), 69–87.

Morsillo, J., & Prilleltensky, I. (2007). Social action with youth: Interventions, evaluation and psychopolitical validity. *Journal of Community Psychology, 35*, 1–16.

Nation, M., Crusto, C., Wandersman, A., Kumpfer, K. L., Seybolt, D., Morrissey-Kane, E., & Davino, K. (2003). What works in prevention: Principles of effective prevention programs. *American Psychologist, 58*, 449–456.

Silverman, J. G., Raj, A., Mucci, L. A., & Hathaway, J. E. (2001). Dating violence against adolescent girls and associated substance use, unhealthy weight control, sexual risk behavior, pregnancy, and suicidality. *Journal of the American Medical Association, 286*, 572–579.

Southern California Injury Prevention Research Center, UCLA School of Public Health, Prevention Institute, & Harvard School of Public Health (2008). *Overview of the UNITY RoadMap: A framework for effective and sustainable efforts.* Retrieved from http://www.preventioninstitute.org/component/jlibrary/article/id-30/127.html

Wekerle, C., & Wolfe, D. A. (1999). Dating violence in mid-adolescence: Theory, significance, and emerging prevention initiatives. *Clinical Psychology Review, 19*(4), 435–456.

Changes in Capacity Among Local Coordinated Community Response Coalitions (CCRs) Supported by the DELTA Program

PAMELA J. COX

Centers for Disease Control and Prevention, Atlanta, Georgia

DANIEL M. FINKELSTEIN, VICTORIA E. PEREZ, and MARGO L. ROSENBACH

Mathematica Policy Research, Inc., Cambridge, Massachusetts

Coalitions are often the means through which communities plan and coordinate services for individuals and address larger environmental issues associated with social problems. Since 2003, the Centers for Disease Control and Prevention (CDC) has supported local coordinated community response coalitions (CCRs) in 14 states to prevent intimate partner violence (IPV) through its Domestic Violence Prevention Enhancements and Leadership Through Alliances (DELTA) Program. Utilizing quantitative and qualitative evaluation data from 2003 and 2006 from DELTA-funded CCRs (N = 59), this article reports on improvements in internal CCR capacity and external supports that can affect the ability of CCRs to prevent IPV. Data are examined through the Interactive Systems Framework for Dissemination and Implementation (ISF) to convey how CCR internal capacity and external supports contribute to the substantial infrastructure needed to effectively address IPV. Family social workers will gain an understanding of the capacities needed by CCRs to prevent IPV, the multiple organizations and systems that support the work of these CCRs, and how they themselves can work to strengthen the capacities of local coalitions that address IPV.

The National Association of Social Workers (n.d.) stated that social work focuses on the well-being of individuals and society by "addressing environmental influences that contribute to problems in living." One problem that affects millions of individuals, families, and society as a whole is intimate partner violence (IPV) (Cox, Ortega, Cook-Craig, & Conway, 2010/this issue). Like many other social problems, the initial occurrence of IPV can be prevented. However, to do so requires the comprehensive, sustained effort of many organizations. To coordinate such efforts, communities often develop coalitions comprising multiple and diverse organizations and stakeholders (Cox, 2005).

Local coalitions that address IPV are often referred to as local coordinated community response coalitions (CCRs) (Cox, 2005). Like other coalitions, CCRs do not usually start off with all the internal capacities and external supports needed to effectively prevent IPV from initially occurring. One internal capacity needed is problem-solving capability that fosters the identification of IPV-related issues and development of appropriate methods to prevent it from occurring (Hawe, Noort, King, & Jordens, 1997). This capacity enables communities to address their own unique IPV issues in a manner that is most appropriate to their communities. To develop this capacity, local communities often need the external support of what are known as "intermediary organizations" (Florin, Mitchell, & Stevenson, 1993), whose mission is to provide funding, training, and technical assistance to local coalitions so that these local coalitions are more effective in their efforts to prevent IPV.

Based on cross-site evaluation data, this article reports on improvements in the internal capacity and external support of 59 CCRs that were supported by the Domestic Violence Prevention Enhancements and Leadership Through Alliances (DELTA) Program of the Centers for Disease Control and Prevention (CDC) from 2003 to 2006. By understanding the internal capacities and external support needed from intermediary organizations by CCRs to prevent IPV from initially occurring, family social workers will be able to identify ways they can work to increase the capacities of and provide support to any local coalition with which they collaborate.

The DELTA Program

CDC initiated the DELTA Program in 2002 to promote the primary prevention of IPV within existing state and local not-for-profit organizations that already addressed IPV by providing crisis services to victims or holding perpetrators accountable. CDC recognized that, although these state and local organizations were already invested in addressing IPV, few of these organizations focused on the primary prevention of IPV. Thus, CDC recognized that it needed to increase the primary prevention capacity of these existing organizations if it was to fund and support these organizations to implement IPV primary prevention efforts through the DELTA Program.

To increase the IPV primary prevention capacity of state and local organizations, CDC established an organizational structure for the DELTA Program that consisted of CDC, 14 DELTA-funded state domestic violence coalitions (SDVCs), and 59 DELTA-funded CCRs operating within the 14 states (Alaska, California, Delaware, Florida, Kansas, Michigan, Montana, New York, North Carolina, North Dakota, Ohio, Rhode Island, Virginia, and Wisconsin). The DELTA Program has had three phases based on its three funding announcements released in 2002 (Phase I), 2005 (Phase II), and 2009 (Phase III). In 2004, the average award to the SDVCs was $291,000, with 75% of each award being mandated for the support of the CCRs.

The DELTA Program defined a CCR as an organized effort representing diverse sectors of a local community that addresses IPV by integrating prevention and intervention strategies and services through increased communication, cooperation, and coordination. Similar to other coalitions, DELTA CCRs are often composed of organizations and individuals who have common interests and work toward achieving common goals (Feighery & Rogers, 1990; Florin et al., 1993). Most DELTA CCRs are not incorporated as formal private or public nonprofit organizations but are informal groups that rely on the commitment of volunteers to operate.

The DELTA Program's efforts to increase the internal capacity of and provide support to CCRs can be understood through the Interactive Systems Framework for Dissemination and Implementation (ISF) (Wandersman et al., 2008). The ISF illustrates how systems and organizations work together and separately to gather and distribute the best available research evidence on how to prevent IPV so that this evidence can be easily integrated practice settings. This framework provides family social workers with an understanding of the multiple organizations, systems, and capacities needed to address environmental influences (e.g., traditional gender norms, social norms supportive of violence, and poverty) that contribute to IPV. Within the ISF, two types of capacity are recognized: general and prevention. *General capacity* is defined as the infrastructure that an organization needs to implement or improve any program, process, principle, or policy (Flaspohler, Duffy, Wandersman, Stillman, & Maras, 2008). This may include strategic plans, fiscal management processes, office supplies and equipment, and leadership. Research suggests that organizations with sufficient general capacity are more able to successfully implement new prevention activities than organizations without sufficient general capacity (Livet, Courser, & Wandersman, 2008).

Within the DELTA Program, *prevention capacity* is defined as the structures, processes, resources, and willingness (i.e., leadership) an organization needs to implement the public health processes included in the DELTA Program's definition of prevention. These processes are (1) reducing risk factors associated with IPV, (2) promoting protective factors that reduce the likelihood of IPV, (3) conducting evidence- and theory-supported prevention planning, (4) addressing risk and protective factors at all levels of the social ecology (i.e., individual, relationship, community, and societal), and (5) evaluating activities. Promoting protective factors emphasizes a health promotion approach (Green & Kreuter, 1991) of encouraging the adoption of behaviors and attitudes associated with healthy intimate relationships (e.g., respect for women and girls). This definition does not include deterrence approaches that are intended to dissuade someone from perpetrating IPV (e.g., educating someone about the criminal penalties) or risk-reduction approaches that are intended to reduce someone's risk of becoming a victim (e.g., self-defense classes).

The DELTA Program's efforts to increase the internal capacity of and provide support to CCRs involve a complex set of activities that occur at the federal, state, and community levels (see Figure 1). At the federal level, the CDC's role in building the general and prevention capacity of state and local organizations within the DELTA Program is as the national synthesis and translation system, the national prevention support system, and the funder of the 14 SDVCs. As the national synthesis and translation

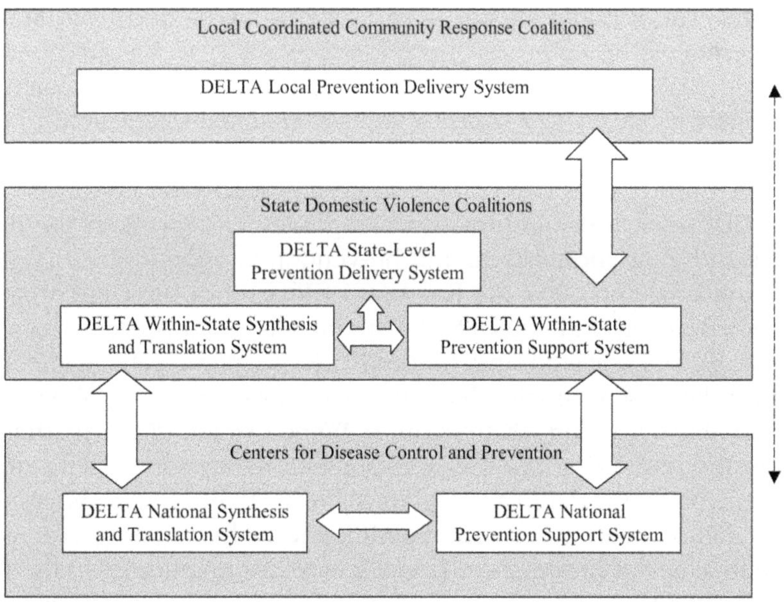

FIGURE 1 Delta Program Interactive Systems Framework, 2002–2012.

system, CDC synthesizes existing research and practice information and translates it to meet the common general and prevention capacity needs of the 14 SDVCs and their CCRs. As the national prevention support system, CDC provides training and technical assistance to SDVCs based on the research and practice material that it synthesizes and translates.

At the state level, SDVCs fund the 59 CCRs and serve as the within-state synthesis and translation system and the within-state prevention support system. SDVCs take the information that CDC provides, as well as other information they gather, and translate this information to better suit their state's unique needs for addressing IPV. Through their state prevention support systems, SDVCs provide tailored training and technical assistance (e.g., coaching and site visits) to their CCRs on various general and prevention capacity topics. Consequently, the external support provided to each CCR is not uniform across coalitions within the same state or across states but based on each CCR's specific needs. Some SDVCs also act as state-level prevention delivery systems when they work directly to prevent IPV at a state level (e.g., by conducting state-wide media campaigns). CCRs, the DELTA Program's local prevention delivery system, receive external support in the form of funding, training, and technical assistance from their SDVCs to build their capacity to implement prevention activities.

Within the DELTA Program, the interactions among CDC, the SDVCs, and the CCRs are bidirectional (Wandersman et al., 2008) and vary in terms of quality, intensity, frequency, or duration (see Figure 1). As capacity building takes place through these interactions, the quality and strength of these interactions can ultimately influence the implementation of primary prevention efforts. The funding stream from CDC to SDVCs and from SDVCs to CCRs determines the nature of these interactions. CDC has frequent interactions with SDVCs (often several times a month), and SDVCs have frequent interactions with CCRs. CDC and CCRs have minimal interaction, to ensure that CCRs look to their funder—their SDVC—for programmatic guidance. CDC relies on the SDVCs to communicate the needs and concerns of their CCRs to CDC so that this information can guide CDC's work as the national synthesis and translation system and prevention support system.

During 2002 and 2003, the first year of Phase I of the DELTA Program, CDC worked closely with the 14 SDVCs to increase their prevention capacity. Then, the SDVCs selected and funded CCRs to participate in the DELTA Program in late 2003. In late 2006, the first year of Phase II, SDVCs added empowerment evaluators (Fetterman & Wandersman, 2005) to their state synthesis and translation systems and prevention support systems, to meet a requirement of the DELTA Program's Phase II funding announcement. These evaluators were to provide training and technical assistance to CCRs on the public health processes, especially evaluation, reflected in the DELTA Program's definition of primary prevention. Empowerment evaluators were not to carry out the prevention and evaluation work themselves. Phase III of the DELTA Program will run from January 2009 to January 2012 and will continue to focus on building the capacity of CCRs to adopt the DELTA Program's public health processes.

To identify changes from 2003 to 2006 in the internal capacity and external support of DELTA CCRs, DELTA Program cross-site evaluation data were analyzed. The general and prevention capacity of the CCRs, as well as changes in the number of prevention activities implemented by CCRs, are reported here. Finally, changes in the external support received by the CCRs from their respective SDVCs are described. Family social workers will gain an understanding of the internal capacities and external support needed by CCRs to prevent IPV and the ways in which family social workers can work to strengthen a local or state coalitions' capacities to prevent IPV.

EVALUATION DESIGN

Purpose of Cross-Site Evaluation

The purpose of the cross-site evaluation was to assess organizational changes among the 59 DELTA CCRs from 2003 to 2006 in four areas: general capacity and prevention capacity, implementation of prevention activities, and relationships with the SDVCs that provided them with funding, training, and technical assistance. As the support provided by the SDVCs to each CCR was not uniform across CCRs within the same state or across states, but based on each CCRs specific needs, the purpose of the evaluation was not to test a hypothesis. The purpose of the evaluation was to assess for improvement or decline in these four areas so that CDC and the SDVCs could adjust their training and technical assistance accordingly.

Sample Selection

The current study uses data from two waves of surveys conducted with CCRs as a part of the DELTA Program cross-site evaluation. The first survey (referred to as the "2003 CCR Survey") was used to identify and document the needs of all CCRs operating in the 14 DELTA states that met the DELTA Program CCR definition. The final sample for the 2003 CCR Survey was 380 CCRs. At the time this survey was administered, CDC and the SDVCs did not know which CCRs would ultimately receive support from the DELTA Program.

The second survey, referred to as the "2006 CCR Survey," collected follow-up data from only the 59 CCRs that continuously received DELTA funding from late 2003 and early 2004 through 2007. No data were collected from the 321 non-DELTA-funded CCRs in 2006. Only DELTA-funded CCRs completed the 2006 CCR Survey to assess changes in the organizational capacity of DELTA-funded CCRs during the early implementation of the DELTA Program.

Survey Administration

The 2003 CCR Survey was administered between February and April 2004 to CCRs in the 14 DELTA states to assess their activities during calendar year 2003. The survey was sent to the chairpersons of 581 CCRs, who worked with other CCR members to complete a single survey for each coalition. The purpose of the survey was to gather information regarding the needs, activities, and successes of CCRs operating throughout the 14 DELTA states so that the DELTA SDVCs could better support their efforts. During the administration, 42 CCRs were removed from the sample because they were defunct or a follow-up telephone call revealed that the CCR did not meet the DELTA Program's definition of a CCR. Of the 539 CCRs that met the DELTA Program's definition, 380 completed the 2003 CCR Survey, for a response rate of 71%. The 2006 CCR Survey was administered between April and December 2007 to the 59 CCRs that had continuously received DELTA Program funding since 2003. All 59 CCRs responded, for a response rate of 100%. In each state, the DELTA Program state coordinator provided hard copies of the survey to the CCR chairpersons, who may or may not have been the same individual who was chair of the CCR in 2003. As with the 2003 CCR Survey, CCR chairs were encouraged to complete the 2006 CCR Survey in collaboration with the local DELTA coordinators and other CCR members. The purpose of the survey was to gather information that the 14 DELTA SDVCs could use to better understand the activities and training and technical assistance needs of DELTA-funded CCRs. These surveys were returned to the DELTA Program state coordinators, who submitted them to Mathematica Policy Research, Inc. for data entry and analysis.

For the CCRs, completing these two questionnaires was a subjective endeavor that required a degree of familiarity with the various aspects of these CCRs that was considered to be beyond the scope of one individual or outside observers. For both surveys, respondents were encouraged to respond to each item in a manner that best reflected the current needs or activities of their CCR, so that future training and technical assistance efforts could be better tailored to meet their needs. Although a subjective endeavor, the research principle of triangulation of multiple sources/perspectives justifies having the CCR chairperson and several other CCR members work together to complete the survey (Patton, 1999). For both surveys, the possibility that some CCRs intentionally or unintentionally overreported in some areas (e.g., capacities and activities) and underreported in others (e.g., needs) exists. However, the evaluation team believes and the literature (Patton, 1999) supports having people with different perspectives regarding each CCR's needs, capacities, and activities participate in the completion of each questionnaire helped minimize this possibility.

Instrument Development

The 2003 CCR Survey instrument was developed in collaboration with CDC staff and the 14 SDVC executive directors and project coordinators, and informed by a literature review on the work of CCRs. The survey assessed topics related to the CCR's background characteristics, organizational structures and processes, technical assistance and training needs, funding, relationship with the SDVC, intervention-focused processes and activities, and prevention-focused activities. Whenever possible, the survey included measures from other instruments, such as the Coalition Effectiveness Inventory (Butterfoss, 1998), which has been used to assess structures and processes of other community coalitions.

The 2006 CCR Survey was based on the 2003 CCR Survey and developed in collaboration with CDC staff and SDVC executive directors, project coordinators, and empowerment evaluators. In the 2006 CCR Survey, items related to CCR intervention-focused processes and activities were dropped and items that assessed CCR primary prevention capacity were added, to reflect the capacity-building priorities under the DELTA Program.

The 2003 and 2006 CCR Surveys were analyzed based on various ISF constructs, including general and prevention capacity of CCRs, CCR implementation of primary prevention activities, and the relationship between the SDVCs and the CCRs they funded. Both waves of the CCR Survey included several questions regarding the general capacity of the CCR: the organizations that were represented on the CCR, implementation of organizational structures (e.g., mission statements or bylaws) and processes (e.g., strategic planning and orientation of new members), and access to financial and nonfinancial resources for CCR activities. The 2006 CCR Survey also assessed challenges faced by CCRs during the early implementation of the DELTA Program.

The 2006 CCR Survey included several questions regarding the CCR's prevention capacity: the presence of a prevention subcommittee, the year in which the prevention subcommittee was established, the degree to which the prevention subcommittee has influenced the CCR's focus on primary prevention, challenges faced by the prevention subcommittee, and resources available for primary prevention work.

In 2003 and 2006, CCRs were asked to provide an open-ended description of two primary prevention activities they had undertaken in the past year, with *primary prevention* explicitly being defined as efforts to "prevent first-time perpetration or first-time victimization, not strategies that intervene after the violence has already occurred." These items were intended to assess the extent to which CCRs were actually implementing primary prevention activities.

Both waves of the CCR Survey assessed the relationship between the CCRs and the SDVCs by assessing the types of interactions between the

CCR and the SDVC (e.g., CCR members attending events sponsored by the SDVC), the CCR's perceived satisfaction with SDVC interactions, and the strength of the CCR's relationship with the SDVC. The recall period for these relationship questions differed between the two surveys from "during the past 12 months" in the 2003 survey to "since you began receiving DELTA funding" in the 2006 survey.

Data Analysis

The data from the 2003 and 2006 CCR Surveys for the 59 CCRs were analyzed using a mixed-method approach that applied quantitative and qualitative analysis techniques. For quantitative items in the survey, descriptive statistics for the general and prevention capacity characteristics of the sample were computed. The McNemar's test was used to test for statistical significance of differences in CCR capacity characteristics across the two waves. In addition, we tested for differences in CCRs' implementation of any primary prevention activities across the two waves using a McNemar's test, which appropriately handled the fact that the same CCRs were surveyed in both years. We tested for differences in the distribution of the number of prevention strategies (zero, one, or two) implemented by CCRs during the two waves using a test of marginal homogeneity.

For the qualitative descriptions of prevention activities, the evaluation team reviewed and coded all of the reported responses to quantify the percentage of CCRs that implemented activities that reflected the DELTA Program's definition of *primary prevention* between 2003 and 2006. The team used the following four categorizations: (1) primary prevention, (2) not primary prevention, (3) vague, and (4) ineligible. An activity was coded as "primary prevention" if it utilized a health promotion approach, meaning the activity promoted skills, behaviors, or gender norms that support healthy intimate relationships. An activity was classified as "not primary prevention" if it emphasized deterrence or reducing victims' risk, increasing awareness of IPV or where to receive services, building capacity for primary prevention (but not actually implementing a primary prevention activity), or implementing intervention activities. Activities were coded as "vague" if there was inadequate detail to determine whether it was primary prevention. Activities that did not refer to IPV or occurred during a different reporting period were coded as "ineligible."

RESULTS

General Capacity

The 59 CCRs continuously supported by the DELTA Program made progress on several measures of general capacity from 2003 to 2006. For example,

CCRs diversified their membership base. Although the membership of intervention-focused agencies was consistently high during this period and the level remained relatively constant, membership of education agencies, funders, media, and adult protective services increased. The percentage of CCRs that reported representation of intervention-focused agencies such as domestic violence victim service agencies, law enforcement/police, prosecutors' offices, batterer programs, health care providers, mental health services community, and child protective services ranged from 76% to 95% in 2003 and from 75% to 100% in 2006. The percentage of CCRs that included representatives of education agencies or schools increased significantly, from 63% to 78% ($p < 0.05$). CCRs also reported significant increases in representation of funders (from 7% to 24%, $p < 0.05$) and adult protective services/elder services (from 41% to 58%, $p < 0.05$). When asked in 2006 about the challenges CCRs faced regarding operating the CCR in general and not related to a specific program or activity, the top three challenges were membership-related, including maintaining momentum (39%), recruiting diverse members (37%), and obtaining member participation (31%).

CCRs strengthened their organizational structures from 2003 to 2006 (see Table 1), as evidenced by increases in the percentages of CCRs with bylaws or rules of operation (from 24% to 44%, $p < 0.05$), written mission statements (from 64% to 85%, $p < 0.01$), written goals and objectives (from 44% to 68%, $p < 0.01$), and written job descriptions (from 19% to 34%, $p < 0.05$). CCRs were more likely to have structures in place that articulated the general purpose and goals of the CCR (e.g., mission statements) than specific structures to support its operations (e.g., job descriptions). The structures that were most likely to be fully implemented in 2006 were meeting minutes (97%), mission statements (85%), goals and objectives (68%), and written vision statements (59%). The structures that were least likely to have been fully implemented were written job descriptions (34%) and organizational charts (15%).

CCRs also strengthened their organizational processes (see Table 1). In 2003, the majority of CCRs had fully implemented only one process assessed in the current study, namely having a mechanism for decision making, such as voting. Three years later, at least one half of the CCRs had implemented five of the nine processes. Moreover, seven of the nine processes assessed in the study showed significant increases in the percentage of CCRs in which implementation had occurred: having mechanisms for decision making (from 51% to 83%, $p < 0.01$), having mechanisms to solve problems or resolve conflicts (from 32% to 53%, $p < 0.05$), allocating resources in an organized and thoughtful manner (24% to 70%, $p < 0.01$), conducting regular strategic or action planning sessions (from 36% to 59%, $p < 0.01$), orienting new members (from 15% to 39%, $p < 0.01$), regularly training new and old members (from 25% to 68%, $p < 0.01$), and ensuring that members complete assignments in a timely way (from 19% to 42%, $p < 0.01$). One process on which

TABLE 1 CCR General Capacity in 2003 and 2006

	CCRs funded by DELTA	
	2003 %	2006 %
CCRs with fully implemented organizational structures		
Bylaws or rules of operation	23.7	44.1*
A vision statement in writing	—[a]	59.3
A mission statement in writing	64.4	84.8**
Goals and objectives in writing	44.1	67.8**
An organizational chart	15.3	15.3
Written job descriptions	18.6	33.9*
Written minutes from meetings	—[a]	96.6
Established effective communication mechanisms	55.9	—[b]
CCRs with fully implemented organizational processes		
Have mechanisms to make decisions, for example, voting	50.9	83.1***
Have mechanisms to solve problems and resolve conflicts	32.2	52.5*
Allocate resources in an organized and thoughtful manner	23.7	69.5**
Use organized methods for evaluating the CCR's effectiveness	18.6	22.0
Conduct regular strategic or action planning sessions	35.6	59.3**
Orient new members	15.3	39.0**
Regularly train new and old members	25.4	67.8**
Ensure that members complete assignments in a timely way	18.6	42.4*
Ensure that members replace their CCR representative if he or she can no longer participate in the CCR	—[a]	42.4
CCRs receiving funding from at least one nonfederal source	28.8	50.9*
CCRs receiving funding from the following sources		
State or local government	25.4	25.4
Private foundation	8.5	22.0*
Member organizations	8.5	22.0*
Fund-raising activities	10.2	28.8**
Other	—[a]	6.8

Note: CCR = coordinated community response coalitions; DELTA = Domestic Violence Prevention Enhancements and Leadership Through Alliances. $N = 59$.
[a]This item was asked only in the 2006 CCR Survey.
[b]This item was asked only in the 2003 CCR Survey.
*Difference is significant at $p < 0.05$.
**Difference is significant at $p < 0.01$.

there was limited activity was the evaluation of CCR effectiveness, which was low in years and did not change significantly over time.

CCRs diversified their funding bases (see Table 1). The percentage of CCRs that received funding from at least one nonfederal source nearly doubled, from 29% in 2003 to 51% in 2006 ($p < 0.05$). State or local government funding was the most common source of nonfederal funding in 2003 (25% of CCRs) and fund-raising activities were the most common source in 2006 (29% of CCRs). In 2006 more CCRs reported receiving funding from fund-raising activities, foundations, and member organizations than in 2003. Moreover, 29% of CCRs received funding from two or more nonfederal funding sources in 2006, up from 17% in 2003 ($p < 0.10$; data not shown).

Prevention Capacity

The majority of CCRs indicated progress in building their capacity to prevent IPV. Nearly all CCRs had an organized structure that was focused on primary prevention; 64% had a prevention subcommittee and 25% reported that the entire focus of their CCR was on primary prevention. Of the 38 CCRs that reported having a prevention subcommittee in 2006, 95% had formed this subcommittee in 2003 or later, which corresponds with the period for involvement in the DELTA Program. When asked how the prevention subcommittee had influenced the CCR's focus on primary prevention, most CCRs with prevention subcommittees reported that their subcommittees strengthened their focus on primary prevention. Of the CCRs with prevention subcommittees, 51% reported that their focus on primary prevention was much stronger and 34% reported that it was stronger because of the subcommittee.

CCRs reported higher levels of membership support for prevention activities not requiring active commitment or participation (e.g., expressing commitment to or knowledge about prevention work) than activities requiring more direct contributions (e.g., committing personnel or financial resources). Nearly all CCRs reported that the majority of their active organizations/agencies were "committed and supportive of primary prevention activities" (95%) or "knowledgeable about prevention activities" (97%); two thirds of CCRs reported that the majority of agencies "committed personnel to primary prevention activities" (68%). Only 17% of CCRs reported that the majority of active agencies committed financial resources to primary prevention activities.

The most commonly reported prevention resources among CCRs included technological resources to stay connected to prevention colleagues (97%; see Figure 2), informal partnerships with agencies with whom they can collaborate on prevention-related projects (95%), and technology to participate in prevention-related conferences or networking sessions (86%). The least commonly reported prevention-related resources were funding for professional development opportunities (29%) and financial resources for projects (19%).

Prevention Activities

CCRs reported significant progress from 2003 to 2006 in applying their prevention capacity by implementing primary prevention activities. The percentage of CCRs that reported that their CCR had implemented at least

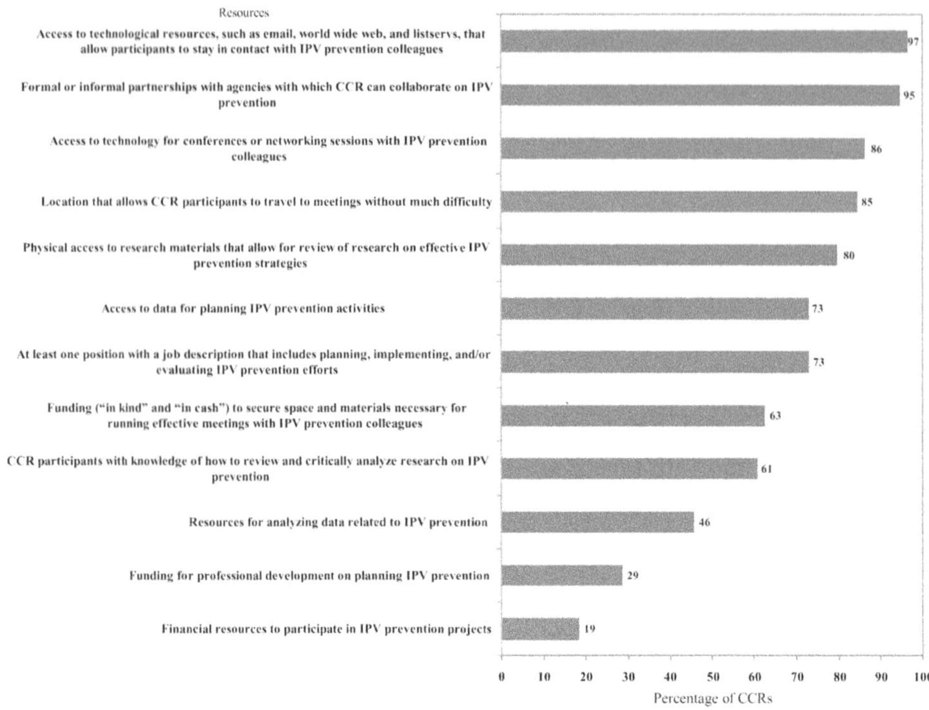

FIGURE 2 Percentage of CCRs that strongly agree or agree that the CCRs' resources related to primary prevention are adequate. CCR = coordinated community response coalition; IPV = interpersonal violence.

one primary prevention activity increased from 32% in 2003 to 93% in 2006 (see Table 2). However, a review of the open-ended description of activities by the evaluation team revealed that many activities reported by CCRs as primary prevention did not meet the DELTA Program's definition of *primary prevention* (80% in 2003 and 16% in 2006). As described earlier, the evaluation team reviewed each activity description and reclassified whether it met the DELTA definition of *primary prevention*.

Focusing only on the activities classified by the evaluation team as primary prevention, there was a 10-fold increase in the reporting of activities classified as primary prevention from 2003 to 2006 (see Table 2). In 2003, only 7% of CCRs reported implementing any activity that was classified by the evaluation team as primary prevention; in 2006, the percentage increased to 78% ($p < 0.01$). The percentage of CCRs reporting two activities classified as primary prevention also increased, from no CCRs in 2003 to 30% of CCRs in 2006. About 60% of the prevention activities focused on preventing first-time perpetration and victimization. Most activities (84%) were targeted at everyone in a population rather than groups that were at elevated risk for IPV perpetration or victimization. The intended audiences were most frequently teenage boys (67%) and teenage girls (55%).

TABLE 2 Classification of CCR Prevention Activities in 2003 and 2006

	CCRs funded by DELTA	
	2003 %	2006 %
CCRs that self-reported implementing at least one primary prevention strategy	32.2	93.2**
CCRs reporting activities that were classified by the evaluation team as implementing at least one primary prevention strategy CCRs that self-reported implementing the following number of primary prevention activities:	6.8	78.0**
0	67.8	6.8**
1	20.3	23.7
2	11.9	69.5
CCRs that were classified by the evaluation team as implementing the following number of primary prevention activities:		
0	93.2	22.0**
1	6.8	47.5
2	0.0	30.5

Note: CCR = coordinated community response coalition. $N = 59$.
**Difference is significant at $p < 0.01$.

CCRs' Relationships With SDVCs

CCRs reported that their relationships with the SDVCs improved from 2003 to 2006. In 2003, 61% of CCRs reported they were very or somewhat satisfied with their interactions with the SDVC; this increased to 76% in 2006 ($p < 0.05$). Moreover, in 2006 approximately 60% of CCRs reported that the strength of the relationship between the SDVC and CCR was much stronger or stronger since the CCR began receiving DELTA funding.

With respect to the type of support they received from the SDVC in 2006, about 90% of CCRs reported receiving materials or resources from the SDVC, 75% reported attending an SDVC-sponsored event, and about one half reported that CCR members attended an SDVC-sponsored event. Only 12% reported that SDVCs attended CCR-sponsored conferences or events. CCRs reported that they were more likely to attend an SDVC event in 2006 (75%) than in 2003 (61%; $p < 0.10$). Otherwise, there were no significant differences in the percentage of CCRs reporting these types of interactions with the SDVC.

DISCUSSION

As coalitions are often the means through which communities address complex social problems like IPV, understanding and developing the internal capacities of and external support needed by local coalitions to effectively address social problems is vital. Family social workers can utilize the results from the current study to inform their work in developing the general and prevention capacities of or providing external support to any coalition with which they collaborate.

Utilizing the ISF to assess changes in internal capacity and external support, the results indicate that the 59 CCRs have increased their general and prevention capacity as well as the number of primary prevention activities they implement. These results also demonstrate that the relationship between the DELTA Program's local prevention delivery system (CCRs) and the DELTA Program's within-state support system (SDVCs) has strengthened since the CCRs began receiving DELTA Program funding.

Between 2003 and 2006, general capacity among DELTA-funded CCRs increased along multiple dimensions, better positioning CCRs to plan and implement primary prevention and intervention activities (Flaspohler et al., 2008). For example, more CCRs had bylaws or rules, written mission statements, written goals and objectives, and written job descriptions. They also strengthened their operational processes, such as regularly training old and new members, allocating resources in an organized and thoughtful manner, and having mechanisms for decision making. These are concrete examples of the types of CCR general capacity that can be increased through strategic investments of time and resources. Knowing that an investment in general capacity is in many ways an investment in prevention capacity and prevention itself, family social workers can promote the development of the capacities listed in Table 1 within coalitions they support.

Prevention capacity among these CCRs also increased during the 3 years of DELTA Program funding. Virtually all DELTA-funded CCRs had developed a prevention subcommittee or focused the entire CCR on prevention. They diversified their membership, especially among schools and other education agencies, funders, and the media. Drawing on the experience of the DELTA Program, family social workers can contribute to building local prevention capacity in their communities by recognizing that IPV is a community problem requiring a coordinated effort of broad community sectors to prevent and develop dedicated prevention committees with diversified membership.

Despite significant progress in building general and prevention capacity, CCRs supported by the DELTA Program still have four key areas of need. The first two areas of need seem to reflect the historical and continued priority of these CCRs and their member organizations to address the needs of victims of IPV and hold perpetrators accountable. The key lesson here for family social workers and others who decide to promote primary prevention within their own communities and coalitions is that integrating primary prevention into structures that have historically focused on intervention activities can be done, but takes time and dedicated effort.

First, the CCRs need to increase their ability to report prevention activities accurately. Although the number of CCRs that could report prevention activities consistent with the DELTA Program's definition of *primary prevention* increased substantially between 2003 and 2006, in 2006 a sizable proportion of CCRs reported activities that were intervention rather than prevention, or their descriptions were too vague to classify the activity as prevention or intervention. Second, CCRs need to increase the active participation of coalition members in primary prevention activities. Although the vast majority of CCRs perceive that their members are knowledgeable about and committed to the coalitions' primary prevention activities, most CCRs reported that their members do not share the primary prevention workload or commit financial resources to primary prevention. Thus, CCRs may need to identify and recruit more members whose priorities are compatible with primary prevention work so that they can create more synergies and leverage more resources.

The third area of need for these 59 DELTA-funded CCRs is funding. Since DELTA Program funding began, more CCRs reported receiving funding from nonfederal sources, such as fund-raising activities, foundations, and member organizations. Nevertheless, funding for primary prevention activities beyond what is provided by the DELTA Program remains a challenge. Few CCRs reported that their member organizations were willing to commit financial resources or that financial resources were adequate to support primary prevention activities.

The final area of need for these CCRs is to increase their ability to evaluate their prevention activities. As most empowerment evaluators were added in the second half of 2006, the impact of their work to date is not reflected in this article. Empowerment evaluators will continue to work with CCRs under DELTA Phase III to build their evaluation capacity through the learn-by-doing process of evaluating one or more of their strategies.

Several caveats affect the interpretation and generalizability of the findings from the current study. First, the data were self-reported by CCRs, and the responses have not been validated by an external source. Second, it is not possible to infer causality. The changes in capacity reported cannot be assumed to be a direct result of the DELTA Program due to the study design. Moreover, CCRs that were selected to receive DELTA funding may have had higher levels of capacity at the outset of funding; thus, some of the changes observed between 2003 and 2006 may be attributed to their readiness for the DELTA Program. Nevertheless, the findings suggest that many changes in CCR capacity occurred since they began participating in the DELTA Program, and it is reasonable to expect that many of these changes would not have happened in the absence of support from their respective SDVCs. Finally, the current study includes only the 59 CCRs that continuously received DELTA Program funding between 2003 and 2007. Thus, these results are not generalizable to the CCRs that did not receive external support from a DELTA Program SDVC.

Family social workers are astutely aware of the importance and power of collective action to ameliorate problems such as IPV. CCRs can provide family social workers with a venue through which to promote collective action to address the environmental factors associated with IPV. However, to be effective in addressing these environmental factors, CCRs need sufficient general and prevention capacity. The development of these capacities often requires the external support of other organizations, such as SDVCs. The 59 CCRs, representing the DELTA Program's local prevention delivery system, have clearly made progress in expanding these capacities. In DELTA Phase III, the CDC and SDVCs will continue to provide external support to these CCRs to build their capacities. Family social workers can utilize the information from this article to guide their efforts in strengthening the general and prevention capacity of CCRs with which they work. They can help build needed capacities through training, technical assistance, volunteering for specific capacity-building tasks (e.g., developing a mission statement or goals and objectives), and fund development. Problems such as IPV are not eradicated quickly, but over time as many small actions eventually have great effect. The actions family social workers take today to strengthen the capacity of their CCRs can help prevent IPV tomorrow.

REFERENCES

Butterfoss, F. D. (1998). *Coalition Effectiveness Inventory (CEI) self assessment tool.* Norfolk, VA: Health Promotion and Disease Prevention, Center for Pediatric Research.

Cox, P. J. (2005). *Community ownership of coordinated community responses to intimate partner violence* (Unpublished doctoral dissertation). University of Georgia, Athens.

Cox, P. J., Ortega, S., Cook-Craig, P., & Conway, P. (2010). Strengthening systems for the primary prevention of intimate partner violence and sexual violence: CDC's DELTA and EMPOWER Programs. *Journal of Family Social Work, 13*(4), 287–296.

Feighery, E., & Rogers, T. (1990). *Building and maintaining effective coalitions.* Palo Alto, CA: Health Promotion Resource Center, Stanford Center for Research in Disease Prevention.

Fetterman, D. M., & Wandersman, A. (Eds.). (2005). *Empowerment evaluation principles in practice.* New York: Guilford.

Flaspohler, P., Duffy, J., Wandersman, A., Stillman, L., & Maras, M. A. (2008). Unpacking prevention capacity: An intersection of research-to-practice models and community-centered models. *American Journal of Community Psychology, 41*(3/4), 182–196.

Florin, P., Mitchell, R., & Stevenson, J. (1993). Identifying training and technical assistance needs in community coalitions: A developmental approach. *Health Education Research, 8*(3), 417–432.

Green, L. W., & Kreuter, M. W. (1991). *Health promotion planning: An educational and environmental approach*. Palo Alto, CA: Mayfield.

Hawe, P., Noort, M., King, L., & Jordens, C. (1997). Multiplying health gains: The critical role of capacity-building within health promotion programs. *Health Policy, 39*, 29–42.

Livet, M., Courser, M., & Wandersman, A. (2008). The prevention delivery system: Organizational context and use of comprehensive programming frameworks. *American Journal of Community Psychology, 41*(3/4), 361–378.

National Association of Social Workers. (n.d.). *Code of ethics of the National Association of Social Workers*. Retrieved from http://www.socialworkers.org/pubs/code/code.asp

Patton, M. Q. (1999). Enhancing the quality and credibility of qualitative analysis. *Health Research Services, 34*(5), 1189–1208.

Wandersman, A., Duffy, J., Flaspohler, P., Noonan, R., Lubell, K., Stillman, L., et al. (2008). Bridging the gap between prevention research and practice: The interactive systems framework for dissemination and implementation. *American Journal of Community Psychology, 41*(3/4), 171–181.

Lessons Learned in Strengthening Systems for Primary Prevention of Intimate Partner Violence and Sexual Violence

PATRICIA G. COOK-CRAIG
University of Kentucky, Lexington, KY

SANDRA ORTEGA
Independent Consultant for Ohio's DELTA and RPE Programs, Columbus, OH

PAT CONWAY
Essentia Institute of Rural Health, Duluth, MN

PAMELA J. COX AND THERESA L. ARMSTEAD
Centers for Disease Control and Prevention, Atlanta GA[1]

The lessons learned from the DELTA (Domestic Violence Prevention Enhancements and Leadership through Alliances) Program and the EMPOWER (Enhancing and Making Programs Work to End Rape) Program can act as a roadmap to guide the next steps of the movement to end the perpetration of sexual (SV) and interpersonal violence (IPV). The introduction of this book argues that the power of prevention systems is that they can eliminate persistent social problems through a sustained, comprehensive, and coordinated approach of a community's network of individuals and institutions. Taken together, the lessons learned in the chapters of this book identify key areas to be addressed to further the work of strengthening prevention systems. Important components to building an effective prevention system highlighted throughout the book are discussed below.

BUILDING A NEW FRAMEWORK FOR PREVENTION PLANNING

The picture that emerges from the work described in this book is one of a group of states that embraced a new way of approaching prevention planning to address the perpetration of sexual and interpersonal violence. This approach, guided by an Empowerment Evaluation (EE) framework (Fetterman, 1998, 2001), was built on the use of a common theoretical basis from which other relevant perspectives were incorporated. From this conceptually sound foundation, the RPE Model of Community Change, states approached their team building in a way that promoted inclusion by using varied and alternative methods for seeking input and organizing their work. They approached their planning processes, capacity building activities and strategy implementation in a data-driven way. This was done not only for the main goal of selecting new prevention strategies, but also for building state and local prevention system capacity. The transformation of prevention system capacity in communities can have longer lasting effects than the implementation of any single strategy, as the transformation changes the ability of communities to select, adapt, evaluate, and sustain strategies over time and as conditions change (Cox, Lang, Townsend, & Campbell, 2010). The discussion below highlights the application of five components of this new approach to prevention planning that permeated the chapters and projects discussed in this book, including use of empowerment evaluation principles and multiple theoretical perspectives, experimenting with strategies for inclusion, engaging in data driven planning, and focusing on capacity building.

The use of empowerment evaluation as a set of guiding principles. Each of the practice articles in this book highlight how EE enhanced their planning and capacity building processes. EE is defined as the use of evaluation concepts as a means of promoting self-determination and improvement (Fetterman, 1994; 2002). The use of an EE framework from the origins of the EMPOWER and DELTA programs allowed for evaluation concepts to be threaded through each stage of the work in which states engaged; not just activities that were labeled "evaluation". As a part of the team building process and prevention plan development, the EE framework acted as a catalyst to help states foster a change in the power structure of the planning process from one that created and disseminated prevention plans to state and local constituencies to one that guided coalitions and health departments to create a plan that is "owned" by community and state planning teams and their constituencies (Conway et al., 2010). Several EE principles were highlighted as especially helpful, *inclusion* (Cook-Craig, 2010); *improvement* (Cook-Craig, 2010); *shared ownership* (Kervin & Obinna, 2010); *democratic participation* (Conway et al., 2010), and *social justice* (Conway et al., 2010).

Operating from an intentional and rich theory basis. The basis for the work of the DELTA and EMPOWER programs is the public health approach (Cox, Ortega, Cook-Craig, Conway, 2010). This approach combines the application of Risk and Resilience theory (see Kantor & Jasinski, 1998; Loh, Gidycz, Lobo, & Luthra, 2005) with the social ecological model (see Dahlberg & Krug, 2002). The combination of those two perspectives allow for the examination of the risk factors for the perpetration of sexual violence and interpersonal violence at the four levels of the social ecology, including at the individual, relationship, community, and societal levels (CDC, n.d.a & n.d.b). In addition, EMPOWER states used the Rape, Prevention, and Education Theory Model of Community Change, which combines Community Readiness Theory (Edwards, Jumper-Thurman, Plested,

Oetting, & Swanson, 2000) and Diffusion of Innovation (Rogers, 1995) to direct the process of mobilizing community partners and planning for the dissemination of SV and IPV strategies using traditional and non-traditional partners in communities (Cox, Lang, Townsend, & Campbell, 2010).

With those common theoretical assumptions guiding their work, states were successful in using a variety of theories to augment various tasks associated with the planning process. To help understand patterns of collaboration among practitioners in communities, Kentucky used concepts from social network theory (Cook-Craig, 2010). North Dakota outlined their use of concepts from feminist theory, Kohlberg's Theory of Moral Development (Daeg de Mott, 2009) and Olweis' approach to bullying (Olweis, 1993) to complete SV and IPV prevention plans (Conway et al., 2010). Undergirding their strategy to employ youth action strategies to prevent teen dating violence, Wisconsin relied on a Health Belief Model (Aiken, Gerend, & Jackson, 2001; Kervin & Obinna, 2010).

Experimenting with strategies to promote inclusion. One of the most difficult challenges in operating from an EE framework is ensuring that participation in the process is accessible and inclusive. The case studies in this book reflect a concerted effort to seek out and test strategies that would overcome barriers for communities and constituencies to participate in the creation of violence prevention and evaluation plans. For example, Cook-Craig, et al. (2010) highlight the use of technology to bridge geographical distance between rural communities and to provide access to literature on evidence-based strategies that may be hard for local programs to access. Perhaps the extent to which capacity building teams vary and test the use of innovative strategies to decrease barriers to participation, the greater the likelihood that EE principles will be reflected. Having greater participation allows the use of local knowledge and selection of evidence-based strategies to become a meaningful part of SV and IPV prevention planning, strategy implementation, and evaluation. In addition, the use of varied strategies may provide avenues for broad discussions on how to combine the use of evidence-based strategies with adaptation processes. For instance, many articles highlight the importance of addressing intersectionality or "the intersections of systems of power (e.g., race, class, gender, and sexual orientation) and oppression (prejudice, class stratification, gender, inequality, and heterosexist bias)" (Bograd 1999, p. 276; see also Crenshaw, 1991; Sokoloff & Dupont, 2005) when promoting the use of specific strategies to respond to violence. The use of an EE framework when engaging in adaptation can ensure that strategies will fit local culture and respond to issues of intersectionality when multiple layers of oppression impact individuals and communities at risk of SV and IPV.

Kervin and Obinna (2010) gave a poignant example of how their decision to implement a youth action strategy in an alternative school opened new avenues for practitioners to gain additional insights into a population vulnerable to violence. Kervin and Obinna show how this became a win-win for those involved, where practitioners were able to reassess assumptions they held about students in alternative schools and the school was able to create successes, which increased their pride in their school community. This was presented as an unintended success and as such, it emphasizes the need to reflect on how the work that is done promotes inclusion or exclusion of populations at risk.

Application of a data driven planning process. Just as the chapters in this book reflect a set of experiences where states embraced the incorporation of theoretical rigor in their work, they also reveal a commitment to the use of quantitative and qualitative data to inform each step of the planning process. The rich nature of the variety of examples of the types of data used is impressive. Qualitative analysis using a multiple case study design was employed by both Conway et al. (2010) and Cook-Craig et al., to allow for systematic reflection on how selected states moved through the process of doing violence prevention planning and capacity building work. In addition, Conway et al. (2010) included an example of quantitative data analysis used in each of their three case studies to demonstrate the variety of ways state prevention teams used data to complete their community assessments. Cook-Craig (2010) demonstrated the use of network visualization techniques to help their state examine variations in how community partners across their state work collaboratively together. Kervin and Obinna (2010) used a mixed methods strategy in which quantitative and qualitative data were used to evaluate the effectiveness of their youth action strategies to prevent violence in high schools. Finally, Cox, Finkelstein, et al. (2010) engaged in a quantitative evaluation to assess changes in capacity of Coordinated Community Response Coalitions (CCR's) as a result of their participation in the DELTA program.

The ability of state and local partners to gather and examine data to inform team composition, community and statewide assessments, strategy selection, implementation processes, and outcomes of their work represents the realization of the EE principle of shared ownership. By taking ownership and responsibility of their data for decision-making and improvement purposes, programs described in these chapters represent a set of experiences in which state and local programs made a commitment to build the capacity needed to make data a focal point in the prevention planning process. The collection, review, and use of data are typically a set of tasks reserved for program evaluators. These chapters, however, give examples of how all stakeholders can participate in and benefit from the use of data.

The importance of building capacity. At their core, DELTA and EMPOWER are programs whose primary goal is to encourage capacity building to prevent the perpetration of violence. DELTA was designed to encourage the development of capacity of local programs to prevent the perpetration of IPV. EMPOWER was designed to encourage the development of statewide capacity to prevent SV. Specifically, states were led through a process in which the intended outcome was a stronger prevention system capacity (for a more detailed discussion on how capacity was operationalized see Cox, Finkelstein, et al. 2010). The intentional aim of promoting greater *capacity* to prevent the perpetration of SV and IPV allowed states to engage in work that transformed the bedrock of how they do their work, such as their resources, data and evaluation capacity, partnerships, leadership, and communication. As Cox, Finkelstein et al. (2010) highlight, the prevention of IPV (as well as SV) depends on our ability to assess gaps in internal and external capacities to do the work needed and strategies to fill these gaps and evaluate progress made. In the DELTA program, state domestic violence coalitions filled the gaps by promoting prevention through training and technical assistance for CCRs across their states (on page 99).

ONGOING CHALLENGES TO STRENGTHENING SV AND IPV PREVENTION SYSTEMS

While this book presents a set of stories that are indicative of a wealth of successes and lessons learned in the two programs, they also point to a number of challenges incurred by each state. Some of the challenges are discussed below.

Learning the Public Health Approach/EE Framework. As noted above, states were thorough and innovative in their identification and application of theory in their work. The states observed, however, that the process of incorporating the public health approach and shifting their orientation to the use of empowerment evaluation principles was at times difficult (Conway et al., 2010; Kervin & Obinna, 2010). The adoption of a process designed to create a system that promotes primary prevention of perpetration of SV and IPV requires dialogue and new conceptualizations of the interplay between intervention and prevention in the fields of SV and IPV (Cox, Finkelstein, et. al, 2010; Kervin & Obinna, 2010). This requires recognition of the importance of both intervention and prevention services and the willingness to challenge existing assumptions of the role of prevention in the field.

In addition, Cox, Lang, et al. (2010) give a detailed example of some of the challenges experienced in New Jersey in understanding and adopting the RPE theory model. While ultimately successful in applying the model, state prevention team members struggled with some components, such as identifying strategies that reflected primary prevention of perpetration across the social ecology. This underscores the importance of taking time to make sure all participants in the planning process can achieve conceptual clarity on theories and models designed to guide their work.

Paucity of evidence-based strategies to prevent SV and IPV. Cook-Craig et al. (2010) discussed challenges in access to literature that details evidence-based violence prevention strategies. An overriding challenge, however, goes beyond providing access to evidence. There remains a lack of strategies to prevent SV and IPV that can be considered evidence-based (Morrison, Hardinson, Mathew, & O'Neil, 2004; Whitaker et al., 2006). This gap in needed evidence elevates the importance of building evaluation capacity and encouraging states and local programs to engage in rigorous program evaluation to assess the effectiveness of strategies employed.

Disseminating lessons learned into the field beyond the pilot. Perhaps the biggest challenge lies in how to effectively and efficiently replicate the successes described in this book beyond the states that piloted this work. Across the chapters, there is a recognition that numerous challenges to obtaining needed resources to do this work exist. In addition, other states may not have access to the type of technical assistance that states in the DELTA and EMPOWER programs received. The successes described here, however, make a compelling case that sustained investment in capacity development is needed, in order for states and local communities to engage in successful efforts in preventing perpetration of SV and IPV. The challenges described here point out much work is still to be done by prevention stakeholders on the ground, program developers, and funders. The prevention planning approach undertaken by the DELTA and EMPOWER programs may offer a promising way forward not just for SV and IPV prevention but other forms of violence as well.

NOTE

1 The findings and conclusions in this chapter are those of the authors and do not necessarily represent the official position of the Centers for Disease Control and Prevention.

REFERENCES

Aiken, L.S., Gerend, M.A., & Jackson, K.M. (2001). Subjective risk and health protective behavior: Cancer screening and cancer prevention. In A. Baum, T.A. Revenson, & J. E. Singer (Eds.) *Handbook of health psychology (pp. 727-746).* Mahwah, NJ: Erlbaum Associates.

Bograd, M. (1999). Strengthening domestic violence theories: Intersections of race, class, sexual orientation, and gender. *Journal of Marital and Family Therapy, 25*(3), 275-289.

Centers for Disease Control and Prevention [CDCa] (nd). Interpersonal violence; Risk and protective factors. Retrieved April 14, 2012 at http://www.cdc.gov/ViolencePrevention/interpersonalviolence/riskprotectivefactors.html

Centers for Disease Control and Prevention [CDCb] (nd). Sexual violence: Risk and protective factors. Retrieved April 14, 2012 at http://www.cdc.gov/ViolencePrevention/sexualviolence/riskprotectivefactors.html

Conway, P., Cresswell, J., Harmon, D., Pospihil, C., Smith, K., Wages, J., Weisz, L. (2010). Using empowerment evaluation to facilitate the development of intimate partner and sexual violence prevention programs. *Journal of Family Social Work, 13*(4), 343-361.

Cook-Craig, P.G. (2010). Using social network theory to influence development of state and local primary prevention capacity-building teams. *Journal of Family Social Work, 13*(4), 313-325.

Cook-Craig, P.G., Lane, K.L., Siebold, W.L. (2010). Building the capacity of states to ensure inclusion of rural communities in state and local primary violence prevention planning. *Journal of Family Social Work, 13*(4), 326-342.

Cox, P.J., Finklestein, D.M., Perez, V.E., & Rosenbach, M.L. (2010). Changes in capacity among local coordinated community response coalitions (CCRs) supported by the DELTA program. *Journal of Family Social Work, 13*(4), 375-932.

Cox, P.J., Lang, K.S., Townshend, S.M., & Campbell, R.J. (2010). The Rape Prevention and Education Theory model of community change: Connecting individual and social change. *Journal of Family Social Work, 13*(4), 297-312.

Cox, P.J., Ortega, S., Cook-Craig, P.G., & Conway, P. (2010). Strengthening systems for the primary prevention of intimate partner violence and sexual violence: CDC's DELTA and EMPOWER programs. *Journal of Family Social Work, 13*(4), 287-296.

Crenshaw, K. (1991). Mapping the margins: Intersectionality, identity politics, and violence against women of color. *Stanford Law Review, 43*(6), 1241-1299.

Daeg de Mott, D. K. (2009). Kohlberg's theory of moral reasoning. In *Encyclopedia of Childhood and Adolescence.*

Dahlberg, L.L., & Krug, E. G. (2002). Chapter 1: Violence—A global health problem. In E. Krug, L.L. Dahlberg, J. A. Mercy, A. B. Zwi, & R. Lozano (Eds.) *World report on violence and health (1-22).* Geneva: World Health Organization.

Edwards, R.W., Jumper-Thurman, P., Plested, B.A., Oetting, E.R., & Swanson, L. (2000). Community readiness: Research to practice. *Journal of Community Psychology, 28*(3), 291-307.

Fetterman, D.M. (1994), Empowerment evaluation. *Evaluation Practice, 15*(1), 1-15.

Fetterman, D.M. (2002). Empowerment evaluation: Building communities of practice and a culture of learning. *American Journal of Community Psychology, 30*(1), 89-102.

Kantor G.K., & Jasinski J.L. (1998). Dynamics and risk factors in partner violence. In: J.L. Jasinski, & L.M. Williams (Eds). *Partner violence: a comprehensive review of 20 years of research (pp.1-43).* Thousand Oaks: Sage Publications.

Kervin, D., & Obinna, J. (2010). Youth action strategies in the primary prevention of teen dating violence. *Journal of Family Social Work, 13*(4), 362-374.

Loh C., Gidycz C.A., Lobo T.R., Luthra R. (2005). A prospective analysis of sexual assault perpetration: Risk factors related to perpetrator characteristics. *Journal of Interpersonal Violence, 20*(10), 1325-1348.

Morrison, S., Hardinson, J., Mathew, A., O,Neil, J. (2004). *An evidence-based review of sexual assault prevention intervention programs.* Washington DC: National Institute of Justice.

Olweis, D. (1993). *Bullying at school.* Malden, MA: Blackwell Publishing.

Rogers E.M. (1995). *Diffusion of innovations (4th ed.).* New York: Free Press.

Sokoloff, N.J., & Dupont, I. (2005). Domestic violence at the intersections of race, class, and gender: Challenges and contributions to understanding violence against marginalized women in diverse communities. *Violence Against Women, 11*(1), 38-64.

Whitaker D.J., Morrison S., Lindquist C.A., Hawkins S.R., O'Neil J.A., Nesius A.M., Mathew A., & Reese L. (2006). A critical review of interventions for the primary prevention of perpetration of partner violence. *Aggression and Violent Behavior, 11*, 151-166.

Index

For Product Safety Concerns and Information please contact our EU representative GPSR@taylorandfrancis.com
Taylor & Francis Verlag GmbH, Kaufingerstraße 24, 80331 München, Germany

www.ingramcontent.com/pod-product-compliance
Ingram Content Group UK Ltd.
Pitfield, Milton Keynes, MK11 3LW, UK
UKHW050756180926
475701UK00007B/1071
9781138841857